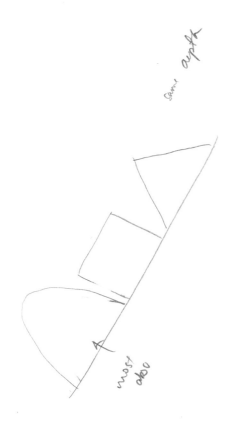

same depth

most abo

Introduction to Medical Imaging
Physics, Engineering and Clinical Applications

Covering the basics of X-rays, CT, PET, nuclear medicine, ultrasound and MRI, this textbook provides senior undergraduate and beginning graduate students with a broad introduction to medical imaging. Over 130 end-of-chapter exercises are included, in addition to solved example problems, which enable students to master the theory as well as providing them with the tools needed to solve more difficult problems. The basic theory, instrumentation and state-of-the-art techniques and applications are covered, bringing students immediately up-to-date with recent developments, such as combined computed tomography/positron emission tomography, multi-slice CT, four-dimensional ultrasound and parallel imaging MR technology. Clinical examples provide practical applications of physics and engineering knowledge to medicine. Finally, helpful references to specialized texts, recent review articles and relevant scientific journals are provided at the end of each chapter, making this an ideal textbook for a one-semester course in medical imaging.

Nadine Barrie Smith is a faculty member in the Bioengineering Department and the Graduate Program in Acoustics at Pennsylvania State University. She also holds a visiting faculty position at the Leiden University Medical Center. She is a Senior Member of the IEEE, and of the American Institute of Ultrasound in Medicine where she is on both the Bioeffects and Technical Standards Committees. Her current research involves ultrasound transducer design, ultrasound imaging and therapeutic applications of ultrasound. She has taught undergraduate medical imaging and graduate ultrasound imaging courses for the past 10 years.

Andrew Webb is Professor of Radiology at the Leiden University Medical Center, and Director of the C.J. Gorter High Field Magnetic Resonance Imaging Center. He is a Senior Member of the IEEE, and a Fellow of the American Institute of Medical and Biological Engineering. His research involves many areas of high field magnetic resonance imaging. He has taught medical imaging classes for graduates and undergraduates both nationally and internationally for the past 15 years.

Cambridge Texts in Biomedical Engineering

Series Editors
W. Mark Saltzman, *Yale University*
Shu Chien, *University of California, San Diego*

Series Advisors
William Hendee, *Medical College of Wisconsin*
Roger Kamm, *Massachusetts Institute of Technology*
Robert Malkin, *Duke University*
Alison Noble, *Oxford University*
Bernhard Palsson, *University of California, San Diego*
Nicholas Peppas, *University of Texas at Austin*
Michael Sefton, *University of Toronto*
George Truskey, *Duke University*
Cheng Zhu, *Georgia Institute of Technology*

Cambridge Texts in Biomedical Engineering provides a forum for high-quality accessible textbooks targeted at undergraduate and graduate courses in biomedical engineering. It covers a broad range of biomedical engineering topics from introductory texts to advanced topics including, but not limited to, biomechanics, physiology, biomedical instrumentation, imaging, signals and systems, cell engineering, and bioinformatics. The series blends theory and practice, aimed primarily at biomedical engineering students, it also suits broader courses in engineering, the life sciences and medicine.

Introduction to Medical Imaging

Physics, Engineering and
Clinical Applications

Nadine Barrie Smith
Pennsylvania State University

Andrew Webb
Leiden University Medical Center

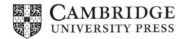
CAMBRIDGE
UNIVERSITY PRESS

CAMBRIDGE UNIVERSITY PRESS
Cambridge, New York, Melbourne, Madrid, Cape Town, Singapore,
São Paulo, Delhi, Mexico City

Cambridge University Press
The Edinburgh Building, Cambridge CB2 8RU, UK

Published in the United States of America by Cambridge University Press, New York

www.cambridge.org
Information on this title: www.cambridge.org/9780521190657

First published 2011
Reprinted 2012

Printed and bound by MPG Books Group, UK

A catalogue record for this publication is available from the British Library

Library of Congress Cataloging-in-Publication Data

Webb, Andrew (Andrew G.)
Introduction to medical imaging : physics, engineering, and clinical
applications / Andrew Webb, Nadine Smith.
    p. ; cm.
Includes bibliographical references and index.
ISBN 978-0-521-19065-7 (hardback)
1. Diagnostic imaging. 2. Medical physics. I. Smith, Nadine, 1962–2010.
II. Title.
[DNLM: 1. Diagnostic Imaging. WN 180]

RC78.7.D53.W43 2011
616.07′54–dc22   2010033027

ISBN 978-0-521-19065-7 Hardback

Additional resources for this publication at www.cambridge.org/9780521190657

''This is an excellently prepared textbook for a senior/first year graduate level course. It explains physical concepts in an easily understandable manner. In addition, a problem set is included after each chapter. Very few books on the market today have this choice. I would definitely use it for teaching a medical imaging class at USC.''
K. Kirk Shung, University of Southern California

''I have anxiously anticipated the release of this book and will use it with both students and trainees.''
Michael B. Smith, Novartis Institutes for Biomedical Research

''An excellent and approachable text for both undergraduate and graduate student.''
Richard Magin, University of Illinois at Chicago

Contents

1 General image characteristics, data acquisition and image reconstruction

1.1 Introduction

A clinician making a diagnosis based on medical images looks for a number of different types of indication. These could be changes in shape, for example enlargement or shrinkage of a particular structure, changes in image intensity within that structure compared to normal tissue and/or the appearance of features such as lesions which are normally not seen. A full diagnosis may be based upon information from several different imaging modalities, which can be correlative or additive in terms of their information content.

Every year there are significant engineering advances which lead to improvements in the instrumentation in each of the medical imaging modalities covered in this book. One must be able to assess in a quantitative manner the improvements that are made by such designs. These quantitative measures should also be directly related to the parameters which are important to a clinician for diagnosis. The three most important of these criteria are the spatial resolution, signal-to-noise ratio (SNR) and contrast-to-noise ratio (CNR). For example, Figure 1.1(a) shows a magnetic resonance image with two very small white-matter lesions indicated by the arrows. The spatial resolution in this image is high enough to be able to detect and resolve the two lesions. If the spatial resolution were to have been four times worse, as shown in Figure 1.1(b), then only the larger of the two lesions is now visible. If the image SNR were four times lower, illustrated in Figure 1.1(c), then only the brighter of the two lesions is, barely, visible. Finally, if the CNR between the lesions and the surrounding white matter is reduced, as shown in Figure 1.1(d), then neither lesion can be discerned.

Although one would ideally acquire images with the highest possible SNR, CNR and spatial resolution, there are often trade-offs between the three parameters in terms of both instrument design and data acquisition techniques, and careful choices must be made for the best diagnosis. This chapter covers the quantitative aspects of assessing image quality, some of the trade-offs between SNR, CNR and spatial resolution, and how measured data can be digitized, filtered and stored. At the end of this chapter, the two essential algorithms for reconstruction of

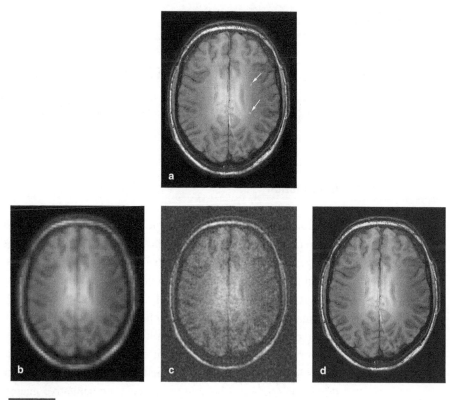

(a) MR image showing two small white-matter lesions indicated by the arrows. Corresponding images acquired with (b) four times poorer spatial resolution, (c) four times lower SNR, and (d) a reduced CNR between the lesions and the surrounding healthy tissue. The arrows point to lesions that can be detected.

medical images, namely the Fourier transform and filtered backprojection, are introduced.

1.2 Specificity, sensitivity and the receiver operating characteristic (ROC) curve

The accuracy of clinical diagnoses depends critically upon image quality, the higher the quality the more accurate the diagnosis. Improvements in imaging techniques and instrumentation have revolutionized early diagnosis and treatment of a number of different pathological conditions. Each new imaging technique or change in instrumentation must be carefully assessed in terms of its effect on diagnostic accuracy. For example, although the change from planar X-ray film to digital radiography clearly has many practical advantages in terms of data storage and mobility, it would not have been implemented clinically had the diagnostic quality of the scans decreased. Quantitative assessment of diagnostic quality is usually reported in terms of specificity and sensitivity, as described in the example below.

Consider an imaging study to determine whether a group of middle-aged patients has an early indication of multiple sclerosis. It is known that this disease is characterized by the presence of white matter lesions in the brain. However, it is also known that healthy people develop similar types of lesion as they age, but that the number of lesions is not as high as for multiple sclerosis cases. When analyzing the images from a particular patient there are four possible outcomes for the radiologist: a true positive (where the first term 'true' refers to a correct diagnosis and the second term 'positive' to the patient having multiple sclerosis), a true negative, a false positive or a false negative. The four possibilities can be recorded in either tabular or graphical format, as shown in Figure 1.2. The receiver operating characteristic (ROC) curve plots the number of true positives on the vertical axis vs. the number of false positives on the horizontal axis, as shown on the right of Figure 1.2. What criterion does the radiologist use to make his/her diagnosis? In this simple example assume that the radiologist simply counts the number of lesions detectable in the image. The relative number of true positives, true negatives, false positives and false negatives depends upon the particular number of lesions that the radiologist decides upon as being the threshold for diagnosing a patient with multiple sclerosis. If this threshold number is very high, for example 1000, then there will be no false positives, but no true positives either. As the threshold number is reduced then the number of true positives will increase at a greater rate than the false positives, providing that the images are giving an accurate count of the number of lesions actually present. As the criterion for the number of lesions is reduced further, then the numbers of false positives and true positives increase at a more equal rate. Finally, if the criterion is dropped to a very small number, then the number of false positives increases much faster than the true positives. The net effect is to produce a curve shown in Figure 1.2.

Three measures are commonly reported in ROC analysis:

(i) *accuracy* is the number of correct diagnoses divided by the total number of diagnoses;

(ii) *sensitivity* is the number of true positives divided by the sum of the true positives and false negatives; and

(iii) *specificity* is the number of true negatives divided by the sum of the number of true negatives and false positives.

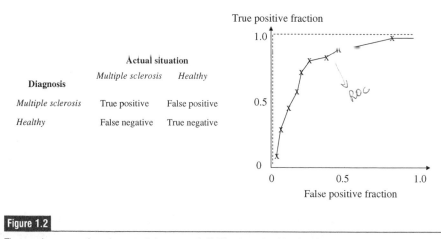

	Actual situation	
Diagnosis	*Multiple sclerosis*	*Healthy*
Multiple sclerosis	True positive	False positive
Healthy	False negative	True negative

Figure 1.2

The receiver operating characteristic curve. (left) The 2 × 2 table showing the four possible outcomes of clinical diagnosis. (right) A real ROC curve (solid line), with the ideal curve also shown (dotted line).

The aim of clinical diagnosis is to maximize each of the three numbers, with an ideal value of 100% for all three. This is equivalent to a point on the ROC curve given by a true positive fraction of 1, and a false positive fraction of 0. The corresponding ROC curve is shown as the dotted line in Figure 1.2. The closer the actual ROC curve gets to this ideal curve the better, and the integral under the ROC curve gives a quantitative measure of the quality of the diagnostic procedure.

A number of factors can influence the shape of the ROC curve, but from the point-of-view of the medical imaging technology, the relevant question is: 'what fraction of true lesions is detected using the particular imaging technique?'. The more lesions that are missing on the image, then intuitively the poorer the resulting diagnosis. 'Missing lesions' may occur, referring to Figure 1.1, due to poor SNR, CNR or spatial resolution. In turn, these will lead to a decreased percentage accuracy, sensitivity and specificity of the diagnostic procedure.

Example 1.1 Suppose that a criterion used for diagnosis is, in fact, completely unrelated to the actual medical condition, e.g. as a trivial example, trying to diagnose cardiac disease by counting the number of lesions in the brain. Draw the ROC curve for this particular situation.

Solution Since the criterion used for diagnosis is independent of the actual condition, effectively we have an exactly equal chance of a true positive or a false positive, irrespective of the number of lesions found in the brain. Therefore, the ROC curve is a straight line at an angle of 45° to the main axes, as shown below.

1.3 Spatial resolution

The spatial resolution of an imaging system is related to the smallest feature that can be visualized or, more specifically, the smallest distance between two features such that the features can be individually resolved rather than appearing as one larger shape. The two most common measures in the spatial domain are the line spread function (LSF) and point spread function (PSF). These measures can be represented by an equivalent modulation transfer function (MTF) in the spatial frequency domain. The concept of spatial frequency is very useful in characterizing spatial resolution, and is explained in the following section.

1.3.1 Spatial frequencies

One familiar example of spatial frequencies is a standard optician's test. In one test, patients are asked to look at a series of black lines on a white background, and then to tell the optician if they can resolve the lines when a series of lenses with different strengths are used. As shown in Figure 1.3, the lines are of different thickness and separation. The spatial frequency of a particular grid of lines is measured as the number of lines/mm, for example 5 mm^{-1} for lines spaced 200 μm apart. The closer together are the lines, the higher is the spatial frequency, and the better the spatial resolution of the image system needs to be to resolve each individual line.

For each medical imaging modality, a number of factors affect the resolving power. One can simplify the analysis by considering just two general components: first the instrumentation used to form the image, and second the quantity of data that is acquired i.e. the image data matrix size. To take the everyday example of a digital camera, the lens and electronics associated with the charge-coupled device (CCD) detector form the instrumentation, and the number of pixels (megapixels) of the camera dictates the amount of data that is acquired. The relative contribution of each component to the overall spatial resolution is important in an optimal

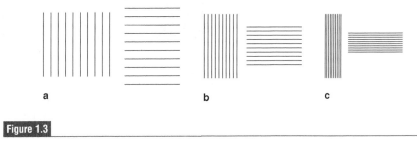

Figure 1.3

Grid patterns with increasing spatial frequencies going from (a) to (c).

engineering design. There is no advantage in terms of image quality in increasing the CCD matrix size from 10 megapixels to 20 megapixels if the characteristics of the lens are poor, e.g. it is not well focused, produces blur, or has chromatic aberration. Similarly, if the lens is extremely well-made, then it would be sub-optimal to have a CCD with only 1 megapixel capability, and image quality would be improved by being able to acquire a much greater number of pixels.

1.3.2 The line spread function

The simplest method to measure the spatial resolution of an imaging system is to perform the equivalent of the optician's test. A single thin line or set of lines is imaged, with the relevant structure made of the appropriate material for each different imaging modality. Examples include a strip of lead for an X-ray scan, a thin tube of radioactivity for nuclear medicine imaging, or a thin wire embedded in gel for an ultrasound scan. Since the imaging system is not perfect, it introduces some degree of blurring into the image, and so the line in the image does not appear as sharp as its actual physical shape. The degree of blurring can be represented mathematically by a line-spread function (LSF), which is illustrated in Figure 1.4.

The LSF of an imaging system is estimated by measuring a one-dimensional projection, as shown in Figure 1.4, with y defined as the horizontal direction. The width of the LSF is usually defined by a parameter known as the full-width-at-half-maximum (FWHM). As the name suggests, this parameter is the width of the particular function at a point which is one-half the maximum value of the vertical axis. From a practical point-of-view, if two small structures in the body are

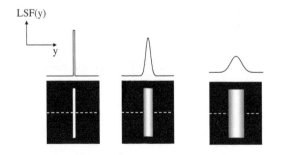

Figure 1.4

The concept of the line-spread function. A thin object is imaged using three different imaging systems. The system on the left has the sharpest LSF, as defined by the one-dimensional projection measured along the dotted line and shown above each image. The system in the middle produces a more blurred image, and has a broader LSF, with the system on the right producing the most blurred image with the broadest LSF.

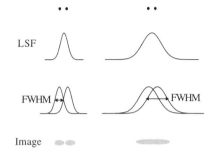

Figure 1.5

Imaging results produced by two different systems with a relatively narrow (left) and broad (right) LSF. In the case on the left, two small structures within the body (top) have a separation which is slightly greater than the FWHM of the LSF, and so the resulting image shows the two different structures. In the case on the right, the FWHM of the LSF is greater than the separation of the structures, and so the image appears as one large structure.

separated by a distance greater than the FWHM of the LSF, then they can be resolved as separate structures as opposed to one larger structure, as shown in Figure 1.5.

The LSF for many imaging techniques is well-approximated by a Gaussian function, defined as:

$$\mathrm{LSF}(y) = \frac{1}{\sqrt{2\pi\sigma^2}} \exp\left(-\frac{(y - y_0)^2}{2\sigma^2}\right), \tag{1.1}$$

where σ is the standard deviation of the distribution, and y_0 is the centre of the function. The FWHM of a Gaussian function is given by:

$$\mathrm{FWHM} = \left(2\sqrt{2\ln 2}\right)\sigma \cong 2.36\sigma. \tag{1.2}$$

Therefore, if the physical separation between two structures is greater than 2.36 times the standard deviation of the Gaussian function defining the LSF of the imaging system, then the two structures can be resolved.

1.3.3 The point spread function

The LSF describes system performance in one dimension. However, in some imaging modalities, for example nuclear medicine, the spatial resolution becomes poorer the deeper the location within the patient from which the signal is received. Therefore, a full description of the spatial resolution of an imaging system requires

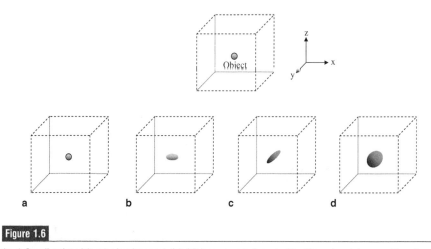

Figure 1.6

(top) Small point object being imaged. (a)-(d) Images produced with different point spread functions. (a) A sharp PSF in all three dimensions. (b) A PSF which is significantly broader in x than in y or z. (c) A PSF which is broadest in the y-dimension. (d) A PSF which is broad in all three dimensions.

a three-dimensional formulation: the three-dimensional equivalent of the LSF is termed the point spread function (PSF). As the name suggests, the PSF describes the image acquired from a very small 'point source', for example a small sphere of water for MRI. Examples of spatially symmetric and asymmetric PSFs are shown in Figure 1.6.

Mathematically, the three-dimensional image (I) and object (O) are related by:

$$I(x, y, z) = O(x, y, z) * h(x, y, z), \tag{1.3}$$

where $*$ represents a convolution, and h(x,y,z) is the three-dimensional PSF. In a perfect imaging system, the PSF would be a delta function in all three dimensions, in which case the image would be a perfect representation of the object. In practice, the overall PSF of a given imaging system is a combination of detection instrumentation and data sampling (covered in Section 1.7), and can be calculated by the convolution of all of the individual components.

1.3.4 The modulation transfer function

The most commonly used measure of the spatial resolution of an imaging system is the modulation transfer function (MTF). This measures the response of a system to both low and high spatial frequencies. An ideal system has a constant MTF for all spatial frequencies, i.e. it exactly reproduces both the fine structure (high spatial frequencies) and areas of relatively uniform signal intensity (low spatial frequencies). In practice, as seen previously, imaging systems have a finite spatial resolution, and the high spatial frequencies must at some value start to be attenuated: the greater the attenuation the poorer the spatial resolution. Mathematically, the MTF is given by the Fourier transform of the PSF:

$$MTF(k_x, k_y, k_z) = F\{PSF(x, y, z)\}, \tag{1.4}$$

where k_x, k_y and k_z are the spatial frequencies measured in lines/mm corresponding to the x,y and z spatial dimensions measured in mm. Properties of the Fourier transform are summarized in Section 1.9. The relationship between a one-dimensional (for simplicity) MTF and PSF is shown in Figure 1.7. The ideal MTF, which is independent of spatial frequency, corresponds to a PSF which is a delta function. The broader is the PSF the narrower the MTF, and the greater the degree to which the high spatial frequency information is lost.

Since the PSF and MTF are related by the Fourier transform, and a convolution in one domain is equivalent to multiplication in the other (Section 1.9.2), the overall MTF of the imaging system can be calculated by multiplying together the effects of all of the contributing components.

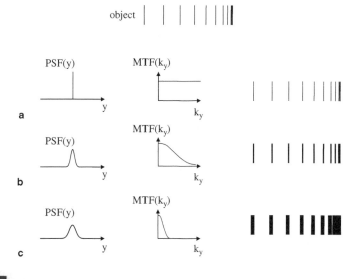

Figure 1.7

(top) The object being imaged corresponds to a set of lines with increasing spatial frequency from left-to-right. (a) An ideal PSF and the corresponding MTF produce an image which is a perfect representation of the object. (b) A slightly broader PSF produces an MTF which loses the very high spatial frequency information, and the resulting image is blurred. (c) The broadest PSF corresponds to the narrowest MTF, and the greatest loss of high spatial frequency information.

1.4 Signal-to-noise ratio

In all measured or recorded signals there is some contribution from noise. Crackle over the radio or on a mobile phone is perhaps the most familiar phenomenon. Noise refers to any signal that is recorded, but which is not related to the actual signal that one is trying to measure (note that this does not include image artifacts, which are considered separately in Section 1.8). In the simplest cases, noise can be considered as a random signal which is superimposed on top of the real signal. Since it is random, the mean value is zero which gives no indication of the noise level, and so the quantitative measure of the noise level is conventionally the standard deviation of the noise. It is important in designing medical imaging instrumentation that the recorded signal is as large as possible in order to get the highest signal-to-noise ratio (SNR). An example of the effects of noise on image quality is shown in Figure 1.8. As the noise level increases, the information content and diagnostic utility of the image are reduced significantly.

The factors that affect the SNR for each imaging modality are described in detail in the relevant sections of each chapter. However, two general cases are summarized here. If the noise is truly random, as in MRI, then the image SNR can be increased by repeating a scan a number of times and then adding the scans together. The true signal is the same for every scan, and so adds up 'coherently': for N co-added scans the total signal is N times that of a single scan. However, the noise at each pixel is random, and basic signal theory determines that the standard deviation of a random variable increases only as the square root of the number of co-added scans. Therefore, the overall SNR increases as the square root of the number of scans. An example from MRI, in which such 'signal averaging' is commonly used, is shown in Figure 1.9. The trade-off in signal averaging is the additional time required for data acquisition which means that signal averaging cannot be used, for example, in dynamic scanning situations.

In ultrasonic imaging the situation is more complicated since the major noise contribution from speckle is coherent, and so signal averaging does not increase the SNR. However, if images are acquired with the transducer oriented at different angles with respect to the patient, a technique known as compound imaging (covered in Section 4.8.4), then the speckle in different images is only partially coherent. Averaging of the images, therefore, gives an increase in the SNR, but by a factor less than the square root of the number of images.

In the second general case, as discussed in detail in Chapters 2 and 3, the SNR in X-ray and nuclear medicine is proportional to the square root of the number of X-rays and γ-rays, respectively, that are detected. This number depends upon many factors including the output dose of the X-ray tube or the amount of

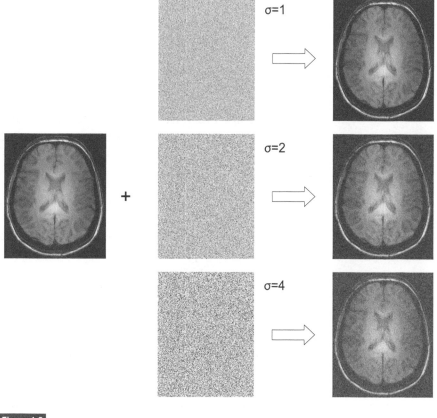

Figure 1.8

The effects of noise on image quality for an MR image. As the standard deviation (σ) of the noise is increased (from top-to-bottom), features within the image become indistinguishable.

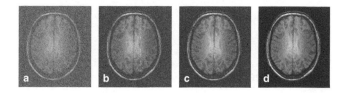

Figure 1.9

Signal averaging to improve the image SNR. (a) MR image acquired in a single scan, (b) two identical scans averaged together, (c) four scans, and (d) sixteen scans.

radioactive element injected and how much radiation is absorbed within the body. The ultimate limit to the SNR is the radiation dose to the patient, with limits which are controlled by various government guidelines throughout the world. X-ray images in general have very high SNR, but for nuclear medicine scans the number of γ-rays detected is much lower, and so the scanning time is prolonged compared to X-ray scans, with the total time limited by patient comfort.

1.5 Contrast-to-noise ratio

Even if a particular image has a very high SNR, it is not diagnostically useful unless there is a high enough CNR to be able to distinguish between different tissues, and in particular between healthy and pathological tissue. Various definitions of image contrast exist, the most common being:

$$C_{AB} = |S_A - S_B|, \tag{1.5}$$

where C_{AB} is the contrast between tissues A and B, and S_A and S_B are the signals from tissues A and B, respectively. The CNR between tissues A and B is defined in terms of the respective SNRs of the two tissues:

$$CNR_{AB} = \frac{C_{AB}}{\sigma_N} = \frac{|S_A - S_B|}{\sigma_N} = |SNR_A - SNR_B|, \tag{1.6}$$

where σ_N is the standard deviation of the noise.

In addition to the intrinsic contrast between particular tissues, the CNR clearly depends both on the image SNR and spatial resolution. For example, in Figure 1.1, a decreased spatial resolution in Figure 1.1(b) reduced the image CNR due to 'partial volume' effects. This means that the contrast between the lesion and healthy tissue is decreased, since voxels (volumetric pixels) contain contributions from both the high contrast lesion, but also from the surrounding tissue due to the broadened PSF. Figure 1.1(c) and Equation (1.6) show that a reduced SNR also reduces the CNR.

1.6 Image filtering

After the data have been acquired and digitized and the images reconstructed, further enhancements can be made by filtering the images. This process is similar to that available in many software products for digital photography. The particular filter used depends upon the imaging modality, and the image characteristics that most need to be enhanced.

The simplest types of filter are either high-pass or low-pass, referring to their characteristics in the *spatial frequency domain*, i.e. a high-pass filter accentuates the high spatial frequency components in the image, and vice-versa. High spatial frequencies correspond to small objects and edges in the images, and so these are 'sharpened' using a high-pass filter, therefore improving the spatial resolution. However, the noise present in the image, since it has a random pixel-to-pixel variation, also corresponds to very high spatial frequencies, and so the SNR of a high-pass filtered image decreases, as shown in Figure 1.10. A high-pass filter is suited, therefore, to images with very high intrinsic SNR, in which the aim is to make out very fine details.

In contrast, a low-pass filter attenuates the noise, therefore increasing the SNR in the filtered image. The trade-off is that other features in the image which are also represented by high spatial frequencies, e.g. small features, are smoothed out by this type of filter. Low-pass filters are typically applied to images with intrinsically low SNR and relatively poor spatial resolution (which is not substantially further degraded by application of the filter), such as planar nuclear medicine scans.

Specialized filters can also be used for detecting edges in images, for example. This process is very useful if the aim is to segment images into different tissue compartments. Since edges have a steep gradient in signal intensity from one pixel to the adjacent one, one can consider the basic approach to be measuring the slope

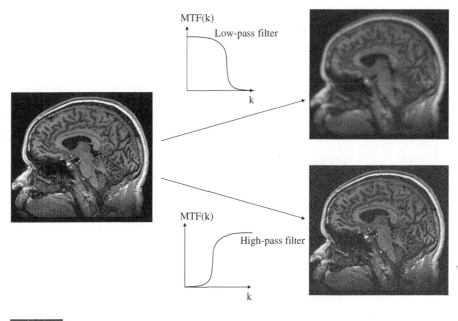

Figure 1.10

The effects of low-pass and high-pass filtering. Low-pass filters improve the SNR at the expense of a loss in spatial resolution: high-pass filters increase the spatial resolution but reduce the SNR.

of the image by performing a spatial derivative. Since edge detection also amplifies the noise in an image, the process is usually followed by some form of low-pass filtering to reduce the noise.

A very simple example of how images can be filtered in practice is the convolution of the image with a specified filter 'kernel'. These can be represented by a small matrix, a typical size being 3×3. In the one-dimensional example shown in Figure 1.11, the image convolution process involves sliding the kernel across the image, multiplying each pixel by the corresponding component of the kernel, and replacing the centre pixel by the sum of these values. The kernel is then displaced by one pixel in the horizontal dimension and the process repeated until the kernel has been applied to all the pixels in this horizontal dimension. In the example in Figure 1.11, the original image has one pixel with a particularly high value (32) compared to the surrounding pixels. After filtering, the difference is much lower, showing the effects of the low-pass, smoothing filter. For two-dimensional filtering, the above process is repeated for the next row of pixels until the whole image has been covered.

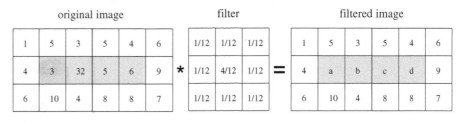

$$a=(1)(1/12)+(5)(1/12)+(3)(1/12)+(4)(1/12)+(3)(4/12)+(32)(1/12)+(6)(1/12)+(10)(1/12)+(4)(1/12)=6.4$$

$$b=(5)(1/12)+(3)(1/12)+(5)(1/12)+(3)(1/12)+(32)(4/12)+(5)(1/12)+(10)(1/12)+(4)(1/12)+(8)(1/12)=14.3$$

$$c=(3)(1/12)+(5)(1/12)+(4)(1/12)+(32)(1/12)+(5)(4/12)+(6)(1/12)+(4)(1/12)+(8)(1/12)+(8)(1/12)=7.5$$

$$d=(5)(1/12)+(4)(1/12)+(6)(1/12)+(5)(1/12)+(6)(4/12)+(9)(1/12)+(8)(1/12)+(8)(1/12)+(7)(1/12)=6.3$$

1	5	3	5	4	6
4	6.4	14.3	7.5	6.3	9
6	10	4	8	8	7

filtered image

Figure 1.11

Numerical example showing the application of a low-pass convolution kernel. The original image is filtered, with image intensities 3, 32, 5 and 6 (shaded) being replaced by a, b, c and d, respectively, in the filtered image. These values are calculated as shown by the terms within parenthesis to give the values shown in the lower grid.

This is a very simple demonstration of filtering. In practice much more sophisticated mathematical approaches can be used to optimize the performance of the filter given the properties of the particular image. This is especially true if the MTF of the system is known, in which case either 'matched' filtering or deconvolution techniques can be used.

1.7 Data acquisition: analogue-to-digital converters

For many years, all medical images were viewed and stored on photographic film. Nowadays, all modern hospitals are in the 'digital age', in which images are acquired and stored digitally. They can be post-processed and filtered to maximize the diagnostic quality, images acquired at different times can be quantitatively compared to determine the effectiveness of a therapy, and images can also be transferred automatically to another hospital if the patient moves location. Irrespective of the particular medical imaging system, the common requirement for producing digital images is an analogue-to-digital converter, which takes an analogue input voltage from the medical imaging system and produces a digital output. With the exception of MRI, the input signals from most medical imaging modalities are not voltages per se, and so must be converted into voltages using an appropriate detector. A general scheme of data flow to produce a digital output is shown in Figure 1.12.

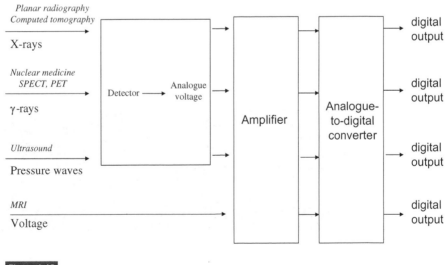

Figure 1.12

Data flow from different medical imaging modalities to produce a digital output.

1.7.1 Dynamic range and resolution

The ideal analogue-to-digital converter (ADC) converts a continuous voltage signal into a digital signal with as high a fidelity as possible, while introducing as little noise as possible. The important specifications of an ADC are the dynamic range, voltage range (maximum-to-minimum), maximum sampling frequency and frequency bandwidth.

The concept of dynamic range is familiar from digital photography and audio devices such as CDs. For example, the dynamic range of a photograph can be expressed as the number of colour levels or the number of graytone levels. The greater the number, the more accurately subtle differences in colour or graytone can be reproduced. Figure 1.13 shows an example of a medical image which is digitized with a different number of graytone levels: clearly the greater the number of levels, the higher the quality of the image. Similarly, for an audio device, the dynamic range describes the difference in sound levels that can be accurately reproduced, from very loud to very quiet. If the dynamic range is too small, then very soft sounds may be too low to be detected.

For an ADC, the dynamic range is measured in bits, and specifies the number of different values that the output of the ADC can have. For an N-bit ADC, the number of different output values is given by 2^N. For example, an 8-bit ADC can have values from 1 to 255 (2^8=256), whereas a 16-bit ADC can give values from 1 to 65535. The difference between these levels is called the resolution, and its value is given by the voltage range of the ADC divided by the number of levels.

256 levels   16 levels   4 levels

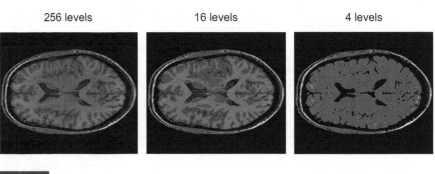

Figure 1.13

Representation of an MR image with a maximum of 256, 16 and 4 graytone levels, corresponding to 8, 4 and 2-bit ADCs. The image quality is already significantly reduced at 16 levels.

Example 1.2   What is the minimum voltage difference that can be measured by a 5 volt, 12-bit ADC?

Solution   There are 4096 different levels that can be measured by the ADC, with values from −5 to 5 volts (note that the maximum voltage of the ADC refers to positive and negative values). Therefore, the minimum voltage difference is given by 10/4096 = 2.44 mV.

Even ADCs with very high resolution cannot reproduce an analogue signal perfectly. The difference between the true analogue input signal and the digitized output is called the 'quantization' error, and this error becomes smaller the greater the number of bits, as shown in Figure 1.14. From Figure 1.14, it can also been seen that the values of the quantization error lie between 0 and $\pm \frac{1}{2}$ of the ADC resolution.

In order to minimize the relative contribution of the quantization errors, therefore, the input voltage to the ADC should be as large as possible, without 'saturating' i.e. going above the maximum value of the ADC (which leads to artifacts). Since the voltages at the output of the various detectors can be quite small, of the order of micro or millivolts, an amplifier is used with sufficient gain to give a signal to fill the ADC.

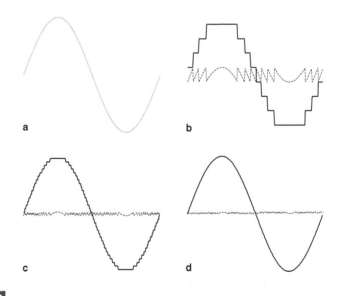

Figure 1.14

Dynamic range and quantization error. (a) The analogue sinusoidal signal which is to be digitized.
(b) The signal recorded by a three-bit ADC (dark line) and the quantization error (dashed line).
(c) Corresponding plot for a five-bit ADC, and (d) a six-bit ADC.

1.7.2   Sampling frequency and bandwidth

The second important set of specifications for the ADC is the maximum frequency that can be sampled and the bandwidth over which measurements are to be made. The Nyquist theorem states that a signal must be sampled at least twice as fast as the bandwidth of the signal to reconstruct the waveform accurately, otherwise the high-frequency content will alias at a frequency inside the spectrum of interest [1;2].

Before digitization, the incoming data pass through either a low-pass or band-pass analogue filter to remove noise components outside the signal bandwidth as shown in Figure 1.15. Acquiring a larger bandwidth than necessary is sub-optimal since the noise level is proportional to the square root of the bandwidth of the receiver. If the measurement bandwidth is less than the range of the frequencies that one is digitizing, the signal outside the measurement bandwidth will be aliased back into the spectrum, as shown in Figure 1.15.

Each particular ADC has a specified maximum sampling rate at which it can achieve its highest resolution: for example many ADCs used for medical imaging systems can sample at 80 MHz with a 14- or 16-bit resolution, but above this rate the resolution drops significantly. If the signal to be digitized has a frequency greater than the maximum sampling frequency of the ADC, then it must be down-converted to a lower value before being fed into the ADC.

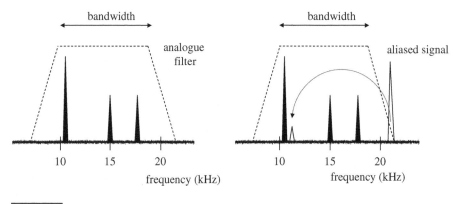

Figure 1.15

(left) A set of signals between 10 and 20 kHz is acquired by setting the central frequency of the ADC to 15 kHz with a 10 kHz bandwidth. (right) If an unexpected signal is present outside the bandwidth at 22 kHz, it is aliased back into the spectrum. Since the signal is partially filtered out by the analogue filter, the intensity of the aliased signal is reduced compared to its true intensity.

1.7.3 Digital oversampling

There are a number of problems with the simple sampling scheme described in the previous section. First, the analogue filters cannot be made absolutely 'sharp' (and have other problems such as group delays and frequency-dependent phase shifts that are not discussed here). Second, the resolution of a 14- or 16-bit ADC may not be sufficient to avoid quantization noise, but higher resolution ADCs typically do not have high enough sampling rates and are extremely expensive. Fortunately, there is a method, termed oversampling, which can alleviate both issues [3].

Oversampling, as the name suggests, involves sampling the signal at a much higher frequency than required by the Nyquist theorem. The process is illustrated in Figure 1.16. Since the bandwidth of the digitized voltage is much higher than the actual bandwidth of the signals of interest, the edges of the analogue filter are placed well away from the actual signals, and the sharpness of the filters is no longer a problem (the other issues of group delays and phase shifts also disappear). A digital filter is now applied to the sampled data to select only the bandwidth of interest: a digital filter can be designed to have an extremely sharp transition. At

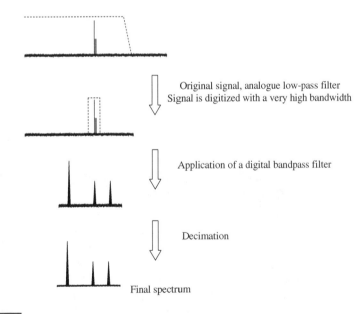

Original signal, analogue low-pass filter
Signal is digitized with a very high bandwidth

Application of a digital bandpass filter

Decimation

Final spectrum

Figure 1.16

An illustration of digital oversampling. The first step is to apply an analogue low-pass filter to remove spectral and noise components at frequencies much higher than the signal bandwidth. The data are sampled at a frequency much greater than the Nyquist frequency. A digital bandpass filter is used to select only the bandwidth of interest. Finally, the process of decimation (averaging of adjacent data points) is used to reduce the quantization noise of the final spectrum.

this stage, the filtered data have N-times as many data points (where N is the oversampling factor) as would have been acquired without oversampling, and the final step is to 'decimate' the data, in which successive data points are averaged together. Since the quantization error in alternate data points is assumed to be random, the quantization noise in the decimated data set is reduced. For every factor-of-four in oversampling, the equivalent resolution of the ADC increases by 1-bit.

1.8   Image artifacts

The term 'artifact' refers to any signal in an image which is caused by a phenomenon related to the imaging process, but which distorts the image or introduces an apparent feature which has no physical counterpart. There are many examples specific to each imaging modality: for example, motion in MRI, multiple reflections in ultrasound, and metal-induced artifacts in both CT and MRI from implants. Recognizing the causes of such artifacts is an important task for the person interpreting the images. Some examples are shown in Figure 1.17: many others are covered in detail in the relevant chapters.

1.9   Fourier transforms

The Fourier transform is an integral part of image processing for all the image modalities covered in this book. In MRI, the signal is acquired in the spatial frequency-domain, and the signals undergo a multi-dimensional inverse Fourier

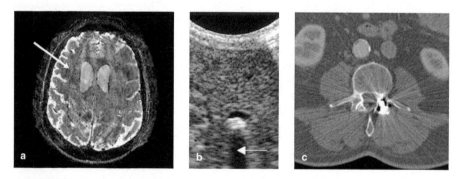

Figure 1.17

Examples of image artifacts. (a) Motion in MRI causes extra lines to appear in the image (arrowed), (b) acoustic shadowing in ultrasound produces a black hole in the image (arrowed), and (c) a metal implant causes 'streaking artifacts' in a CT image.

transform to produce the image. In CT, SPECT and PET, filtered backprojection algorithms are implemented using Fourier transforms. In ultrasonic imaging, spectral Doppler plots are the result of Fourier transformation of the time-domain demodulated Doppler signals. This section summarizes the basis mathematics and properties of the Fourier transform, with emphasis on those properties relevant to the imaging modalities covered.

1.9.1 Fourier transformation of time- and spatial frequency-domain signals

The forward Fourier transform of a time-domain signal, s(t), is given by:

$$S(f) = \int_{-\infty}^{\infty} s(t)e^{-j2\pi ft}dt. \tag{1.7}$$

The inverse Fourier transform of a frequency-domain signal, S(f), is given by:

$$s(t) = \frac{1}{2\pi} \int_{-\infty}^{\infty} S(f)e^{+j2\pi ft}df. \tag{1.8}$$

The forward Fourier transform of a spatial-domain signal, $\rho(x)$, has the form:

$$S(k) = \int_{-\infty}^{\infty} s(x)e^{-j2\pi k_x x}dx. \tag{1.9}$$

The corresponding inverse Fourier transform of a spatial frequency-domain signal, S(k), is given by:

$$s(x) = \int_{-\infty}^{\infty} S(k)e^{+j2\pi k_x x}dk. \tag{1.10}$$

Some useful Fourier-pairs are shown in Figure 1.18: each of the particular functions occurs in multiple instances in the medical imaging modalities covered here.

In imaging, signals are clearly often acquired in more than one dimension, and image reconstruction then requires multi-dimensional Fourier transformation. For example, MRI intrinsically acquires two-dimensional k-space data, for which the Fourier pairs are given by:

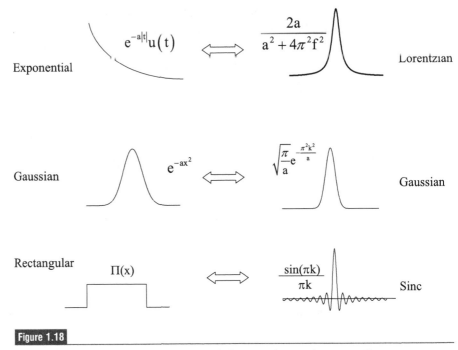

Figure 1.18

Three Fourier transform pairs commonly used in image and spectral reconstruction.

$$S(k_x, k_y) = \int_{-\infty}^{\infty} \int_{-\infty}^{\infty} s(x, y) e^{-j2\pi(k_x x + k_y y)} dx dy, \qquad (1.11)$$

$$s(x, y) = \int_{-\infty}^{\infty} \int_{-\infty}^{\infty} S(k_x, k_y) e^{+j2\pi(k_x x + k_y y)} dk_x dk_y. \qquad (1.12)$$

For three-dimensional MRI data acquisition, a corresponding three-dimensional inverse Fourier transform from k-space to the spatial domain is required. These higher-dimension Fourier transforms are typically implemented as sequential one-dimensional transforms along the respective dimensions. For example, this means that a two-dimensional Fourier transform of a function f(x,y) can be implemented by first carrying out a one-dimensional Fourier transform along the x-axis, and then a second Fourier transform along the y-axis. Highly efficient computational algorithms make the Fourier transform one of the quickest mathematical transforms to perform.

1.9.2 Useful properties of the Fourier transform

In order to understand many aspects of medical imaging, both in terms of the spatial resolution inherent to the particular imaging modality and also the effects of image post-processing, a number of mathematical properties of the Fourier transform are very useful. The most relevant examples are listed below, with specific examples from the imaging modalities covered in this book.

(a) Linearity. The Fourier transform of two additive functions is additive:

$$
\begin{aligned}
as_1(t) + bs_2(t) &\Leftrightarrow aS_1(f) + bS_2(f) \quad, \\
aS_1(x) + bS_2(x) &\Leftrightarrow as_1(k_x) + bs_2(k_x)
\end{aligned}
\tag{1.13}
$$

where $\Leftrightarrow$ represents forward Fourier transformation from left-to-right, and the inverse Fourier transform from right-to-left. This theorem shows that when the acquired signal is, for example, the sum of a number of different sinusoidal functions, each with a different frequency and different amplitude, then the relative amplitudes of these components are maintained when the data are Fourier transformed, as shown in Figure 1.19.

(b) Convolution. If two signals are multiplied together, then the signal in the Fourier domain is given by the convolution of the two individual Fourier transformed components, e.g.

$$
\begin{aligned}
s_1(t)s_2(t) &\Leftrightarrow S_1(f) * S_2(f) \quad, \\
s_1(k_x)s_2(k_x) &\Leftrightarrow S_1(x) * S_2(x)
\end{aligned}
\tag{1.14}
$$

where $*$ represents a convolution. This relationship is shown in Figure 1.20. The convolution, $f(x)$, of two functions $p(x)$ and $q(x)$ is defined as:

$$
f(x) = p(x) * q(x) = \int_{-\infty}^{\infty} p(x - \tau)q(\tau)d\tau.
\tag{1.15}
$$

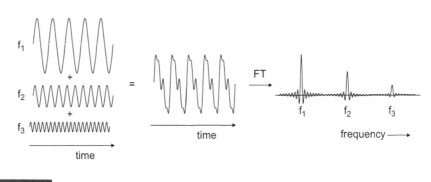

Figure 1.19

A time-domain signal (centre) is composed of three different time-domain signals (left). The Fourier transformed frequency spectrum (right) produces signals for each of the three frequencies with the same amplitudes as in the time-domain data.

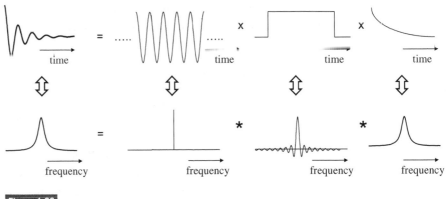

Figure 1.20

The correspondence between multiplication in one domain (time at the top) with convolution in the corresponding Fourier domain (frequency at the bottom). The time-domain signal at the top left can be represented as an infinitely long sine wave multiplied by a finite sampling period (rectangle) and an exponential function. Examples of this type of function are an MR signal or an ultrasound pulse. In the frequency domain, the Lorenzian function (bottom left) is given by the convolution of a delta function, a sinc function and another Lorenzian function which are the Fourier transforms of the corresponding time-domain functions.

In general, the image can be represented by the actual object convolved with the PSF for the particular imaging modality used. Three examples of convolution covered in this book are the effects of a finite beamwidth in ultrasound imaging, geometric unsharpness in X-ray imaging and short T_2 values in MRI. Convolution is also an integral part of image filtering and backprojection algorithms.

(c) Scaling law. If either a time-domain or spatial-domain signal is scaled by a factor b in that particular domain, i.e. stretched or compressed, then its Fourier transform is scaled by the inverse factor, i.e.:

$$s(bt) \Leftrightarrow \frac{1}{|b|} S\left(\frac{f}{b}\right)$$

$$s(bx) \Leftrightarrow \frac{1}{|b|} S\left(\frac{k_x}{b}\right).$$

(1.16)

There are numerous examples covered in this book. Already outlined is the relationship between the PSF and MTF, and the LSF and one-dimensional MTF. Since the parameters are related by a Fourier transform the broader the LSF, for example, the narrower the MTF, and vice-versa, as shown in Figure 1.21.

1.10 Backprojection, sinograms and filtered backprojection

Reconstruction of a two-dimensional image from a series of one-dimensional projections is required for CT, SPECT and PET. A large number of one-

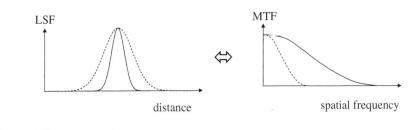

LSF

MTF

distance

spatial frequency

Figure 1.21

The relationship between the LSF and MTF of an imaging system is governed by the Fourier scaling law, in which a broad function in one domain corresponds to a narrow function in the other.

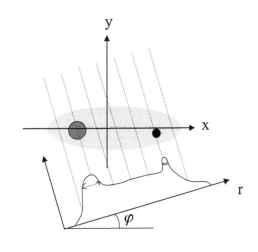

Figure 1.22

The object being imaged is represented as f(x,y) where x and y represent the image coordinates. In this example, higher values of f(x,y) are represented by darker colours. The projection plots the intensity of the projection as a function of r: therefore, the highest values correspond to lines passing through the darker disk-shaped areas.

dimensional projections, p_1, p_2....p_n, are acquired with the detector oriented at different angles with respect to the object, as shown in Figure 1.22. The particular 'image' that one is trying to reconstruct depends upon the imaging modality, i.e. in CT the image corresponds to Hounsfield units (related to the X-ray attenuation coefficient), in SPECT and PET the image represents the biodistribution of the injected radioactive agent. If one considers a single slice through the patient, the relevant parameter in the patient can be expressed mathematically as a function f(x,y), in which the spatially-dependent values of f correspond to the distribution of radiopharmaceutical in SPECT or PET, or attenuation coefficients in X-ray CT. In general, the detector is at an angle of φ degrees to the x-axis for a particular measurement, with φ having values between 0 and 360°. The measured projection at every angle φ is denoted by p(r,φ).

1.10.1 Backprojection

After all of the projections have been acquired, image reconstruction using back-projection assigns an equal weighting to all of the pixels which contribute to each projection. This process is repeated for all of the projections, and the pixel intensities are summed to give the reconstructed image. An example is shown in Figure 1.23. The object consists of a simple cylinder with uniform intensity throughout the disk and zero intensity outside the disk. Projection p_1 is acquired at an angle $\varphi=0°$, projection p_2 at $\varphi=45°$, p_3 at $\varphi=90°$ and so on up to p_8. The process of backprojection assigns an equal weight to all pixels in the reconstructed image for each projection, as shown in Figure 1.23(b). Summation of each individual image gives the result in Figure 1.23(c), which is the backprojected image.

If the object is represented by f(x,y) the reconstructed image is given the symbol $\hat{f}(x, y)$, where the circumflex represents the estimated image, and is given by:

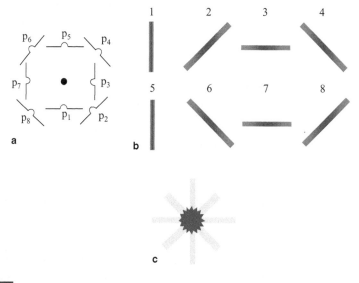

a   **b**   **c**

Figure 1.23

The process of backprojection. (a) From a small round object with uniform signal intensity, eight projections are obtained with angular increments of 45°. The eight projections are shown in (b) with the dark areas corresponding to the highest signal intensity. (c) The process of backprojection involves summation of the images shown in (b). A significant 'star artifact' is visible due to the small number of projections.

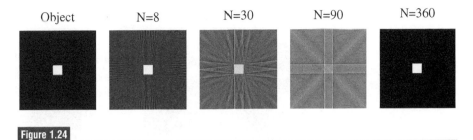

Figure 1.24

The effect of a different number of projections (N) on the backprojected image. The object is a square of uniform signal intensity (far left). With eight projections there is significant signal in areas far away from the object. As the number of projections increases the reconstruction improves, with a perfectly usable reconstruction with 90 projections and an almost perfect reconstruction with 360 projections.

$$\hat{f}(x, y) = \sum_{j=1}^{n} p(r, \varphi_j) d\varphi, \qquad (1.17)$$

where n is the number of projections. Clearly, an important data acquisition parameter is the number of projections which are acquired. If too few projections are acquired, then significant image artifacts occur in data reconstruction: Figure 1.24 shows examples of these so-called 'streak' artifacts.

1.10.2 Sinograms

A common method of displaying projection data is a sinogram, in which the projections are plotted as a function of the angle φ. In order to reduce the dimensionality of the plot the projections are plotted with the signal amplitude represented by the brightness of the sinogram, with a high amplitude corresponding to a bright pixel, and a low amplitude to a dark pixel. As shown in Figure 1.25, sinograms can be used to detect the presence of patient motion, which is visible as a signal discontinuity. Such motions can cause severe artifacts in the reconstructed images.

1.10.3 Filtered backprojection

The process of backprojection as described up to now has an inherent problem in that it results in signal intensity outside the actual object, as shown in Figures 1.23 and 1.24. Although this effect can be reduced by increasing the number of projections that are acquired and processed, use of even a very large number of projections leads to some image blurring. This effect is well-understood, and mathematical analysis shows that applying an appropriate filter function to each projection before backprojection can reduce this blurring [4]. The filter is applied via convolution: the effects on a very simple projection are shown in Figure 1.26.

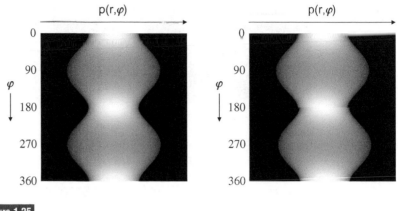

Examples of sinograms from an object which does not move during the scan (left) and which moves roughly half-way through the scan (right), the motion being seen as a displacement in the sinogram.

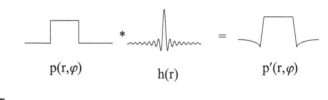

The effect of convolving a projection p(r,φ) with the spatial filter function h(r). The negative lobe in the filtered projection minimizes the 'star artifact' in the reconstructed image.

Intuitively, one can see that the negative lobe introduced around the edges of the projection will cancel out the unwanted positive 'blurring' signal around the edge of the object. From a practical point-of-view, it is important that the process of filtered backprojection be as computationally efficient as possible, since real-time processing of medical images allows interactive image planning while the patient is in the scanner. As described so far, the projection is filtered in the spatial domain, and the resulting filtered projection, $p'(r,\varphi)$, can be represented as:

$$p'(r, \varphi) = p(r, \varphi) * h(r). \qquad (1.18)$$

Since the mathematical process of convolution is computationally intensive and therefore slow, in practice filtered backprojection is carried out in the spatial frequency-domain using fast Fourier transform methods. Convolution in the spatial domain is equivalent to multiplication in the spatial frequency-domain, and multiplication can be performed much faster than convolution. Each projection p(r,φ) is Fourier transformed along the r-dimension to give P(k,φ), and then P(k,φ) is multiplied by H(k), the Fourier transform of h(r), to give P′(k,φ):

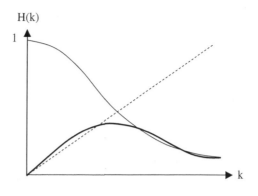

H(k)

k

Figure 1.27

Functions used for filtered backprojection. The Ram-Lak filter [4] (dotted line) represents a high-pass filter, a Hamming function (thin line) is a low-pass filter, and the combination of the two (thick line) produces a band-pass filter.

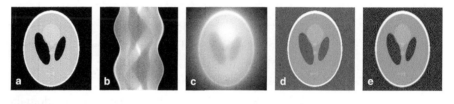

Figure 1.28

The process of filtered backprojection. (a) The Shepp–Logan phantom. (b) The sinogram produced from the Shepp–Logan phantom using 180 projections. (c) Image reconstructed using simple backprojection with no filtering. The image has very high SNR but shows significant blurring. (d) The image reconstructed using filtered backprojection with a Ram–Lak filter applied. The sharp edges in the phantom are well-represented, but the SNR is reduced significantly. (e) Reconstruction with a band-pass filter, shown in Figure 1.27, gives a good representation of the object.

$$P'(k, \varphi) = P(k, \varphi) H(k). \tag{1.19}$$

The filtered projections, $P'(k,\varphi)$, are inverse Fourier transformed back into the spatial-domain, and backprojected to give the final image, $\hat{f}(x, y)$:

$$\hat{f}(x, y) = \sum_{j=1}^{n} F^{-1}\{P'(k, \varphi_j)\} d\varphi. \tag{1.20}$$

where F^{-1} represents an inverse Fourier transform.

The general form of h(r) is shown in Figure 1.26, and various examples of H(k) in the spatial frequency-domain are shown in Figure 1.27.

The effects of filtered backprojection can be seen in Figure 1.28, which uses a Shepp-Logan phantom. This is an object which contains both large and small features, and is very commonly used in assessing image reconstruction algorithms.

The various shapes represent different features within the brain, including the skull, ventricles and several small features either overlapping other structures or placed close together.

Exercises

Specificity, sensitivity and the ROC

1.1 In a patient study for a new test for multiple sclerosis (MS), 32 of the 100 patients studied actually have MS. For the data given below, complete the two-by-two matrices and construct an ROC. The number of lesions (50, 40, 30, 20 or 10) corresponds to the threshold value for designating MS as the diagnosis.

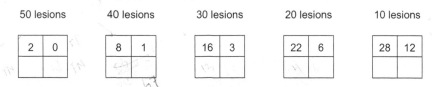

| 50 lesions | 40 lesions | 30 lesions | 20 lesions | 10 lesions |

| 2 | 0 | 8 | 1 | 16 | 3 | 22 | 6 | 28 | 12 |

1.2 Choose a medical condition and suggest a clinical test which would have:
   (a) High sensitivity but low specificity;
   (b) Low sensitivity but high specificity.

1.3. What does an ROC curve that lies below the random line suggest? Could this be diagnostically useful?

Spatial resolution

1.4 For the one-dimensional objects O(x) and PSFs h(x) shown in Figure 1.29, draw the resulting projections I(x). Write down whether each object contains

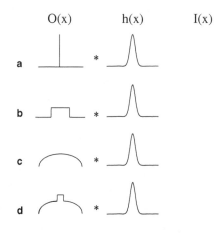

O(x)   h(x)   I(x)

a

b

c

d

Figure 1.29

See Exercise 1.4.

high, low or both spatial frequencies, and which is affected most by the action of h(x).

1.5 Show mathematically that the FWHM of a Gaussian function is given by:

$$FWHM = \left(2\sqrt{2\ln 2}\right)\sigma \cong 2.36\sigma.$$

1.6 Plot the MTF on a single graph for each of the convolution filters shown below.

1	1	1
1	4	1
1	1	1

1	1	1
1	12	1
1	1	1

1	1	1
1	1	1
1	1	1

1.7 What type of filter is represented by the following kernel?

1	0	-1
1	0	-1
1	0	-1

1.8 Using the filter in Exercise 1.7 calculate the filtered image using the original image from Figure 1.11.

Data acquisition

1.9 An ultrasound signal is digitized using a 16-bit ADC at a sampling rate of 3 MHz. If the image takes 20 ms to acquire, how much data (in Mbytes) is there in each ultrasound image. If images are acquired for 20 s continuously, what is the total data output of the scan?

1.10 If a signal is digitized at a sampling rate of 20 kHz centred at 10 kHz, at what frequency would a signal at 22 kHz appear?

1.11 A signal is sampled every 1 ms for 20 ms, with the following actual values of the analogue voltage at successive sampling times. Plot the values of the voltage recorded by a 5 volt, 4-bit ADC assuming that the noise level is much lower than the signal and so can be neglected. On the same graph, plot the quantization error.

p16-17

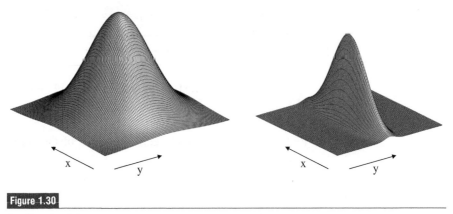

Figure 1.30

See Exercise 1.14.

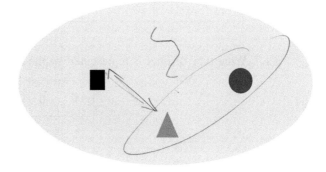

Figure 1.31

See Exercise 1.16.

Signal(volts) = $-4.3, +1.2, -0.6, -0.9, +3.4, -2.7, +4.3, +0.1, -3.2,$ $-4.6, +1.8, +3.6, +2.4, -2.7, +0.5, -0.5, -3.7, +2.1, -4.1, -0.4$

1.12 Using the same signal as in exercise 1.11, plot the values of the voltage and the quantization error recorded by a 5 volt, 8-bit ADC.

Fourier transforms

1.13 In Figure 1.20 plot the time and frequency domain signals for the case where the sampling time becomes very short.

1.14 Figure 1.30 shows two different two-dimensional PSFs in the (x,y) spatial domain. Draw the corresponding two-dimensional MTFs in the (k_x, k_y) spatial frequency dimension, and plot separately the one-dimensional MTF vs. k_x and MTF vs. k_y.

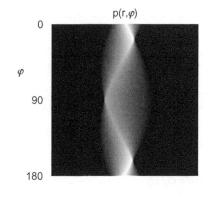

Figure 1.32

See Exercise 1.17.

Backprojection

1.15 For Figure 1.25, suggest one possible shape that could have produced the sinogram.

1.16 For the object shown in Figure 1.31: (a) draw the projections at angles of 0, 45, 90, and 135°, and (b) draw the sinogram from the object. Assume that a dark area corresponds to an area of high signal.

1.17 A scan is taken of a patient, and an area of radioactivity is found. The sinogram is shown in Figure 1.32. Assuming that the radioactivity is uniform within the targeted area, what is one possible shape of the area of radioactivity?

References

[1] Shannon CE. Communication in the presence of noise. *Proc Inst Radio Engineers* 1949;**37**, 10–21.

[2] Nyquist H. Certain topics in telegraph transmission theory. *Trans AIEE* 1928;**47**, 617–44.

[3] Ritchie CR, Candy JC and Ninke WH. Interpolative digital-to-analog converters. *IEEE Trans Communications* 1974;Com-22, 1797–806.

[4] Ramachandran GN and Lakshminarayanan V. Three-dimensional reconstruction from radiographs and electron micrographs: applications of convolutions instead of Fourier transforms. *Proc Natl Acad Sci USA* 1971;**68**, 2236–40.

2 X-ray planar radiography and computed tomography

2.1 Introduction

X-ray planar radiography is one of the mainstays of a radiology department, providing a first 'screening' for both acute injuries and suspected chronic diseases. Planar radiography is widely used to assess the degree of bone fracture in an acute injury, the presence of masses in lung cancer/emphysema and other airway pathologies, the presence of kidney stones, and diseases of the gastrointestinal (GI) tract. Depending upon the results of an X-ray scan, the patient may be referred for a full three-dimensional X-ray computed tomography (CT) scan for more detailed diagnosis.

The basis of both planar radiography and CT is the differential absorption of X-rays by various tissues. For example, bone and small calcifications absorb X-rays much more effectively than soft tissue. X-rays generated from a source are directed towards the patient, as shown in Figure 2.1(a). X-rays which pass through the patient are detected using a solid-state flat panel detector which is placed just below the patient. The detected X-ray energy is first converted into light, then into a voltage and finally is digitized. The digital image represents a two-dimensional projection of the tissues lying between the X-ray source and the detector. In addition to being absorbed, X-rays can also be scattered as they pass through the body, and this gives rise to a background signal which reduces the image contrast. Therefore, an 'anti-scatter grid', shown in Figure 2.1(b), is used to ensure that only X-rays that pass directly through the body from source-to-detector are recorded. An example of a two-dimensional planar X-ray is shown in Figure 2.1(c). There is very high contrast, for example, between the bones (white) which absorb X-rays, and the lung tissue (dark) which absorbs very few X-rays.

There are a number of specialized applications of radiography which require related but modified instrumentation. X-ray fluoroscopy is a technique in which images are continuously acquired to study, for example, the passage of an X-ray contrast agent through the GI tract. Digital mammography uses much lower X-ray energies than standard X-ray scans, and is used to obtain images with much finer resolution than standard planar radiography. Digital subtraction

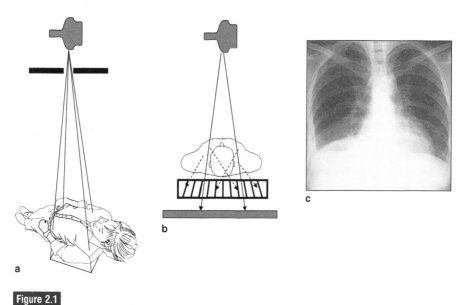

Figure 2.1

(a) The set-up for planar radiography. The X-ray beam from the tube is collimated, passes through the patient, and forms an image on the digital detector placed below the patient. (b) An anti-scatter grid is placed directly in front of the detector to reduce the contribution from scattered X-rays in order to increase the image contrast. (c) An example of a planar radiograph through the chest. The bones attenuate X-rays to a much greater degree than the soft tissue of the lungs, and appear bright on the image.

angiography is a technique which acquires images of the vasculature at extremely high resolution.

For many clinical diagnoses, it is necessary to acquire a full three-dimensional image from a particular region of the body. For head trauma patients, for example, the location and size of the trauma must be determined very accurately. For imaging of the liver and surrounding organs, a two-dimensional planar radiograph would have too much overlap from the different tissues to be useful. The basic principle of CT is shown in Figure 2.2, together with a photograph of a modern multi-detector helical scanner. The X-ray source and a bank of X-ray detectors are rotated in synchrony around the patient. The rotation speed is high, with one revolution taking less than a second. A series of one-dimensional projections is acquired during the rotation, and these are then reconstructed to form a two-dimensional image. The third dimension is acquired by moving the patient in a horizontal direction while the images are being acquired, and also by having not just one but many detector rows (currently up to 320) in the horizontal direction. Using this type of state-of-the-art multi-detector helical CT scanner, very high resolution images of large volume can be acquired very rapidly. Figure 2.2 also shows an example of a three-dimensional image of the heart, with exquisite visualization of

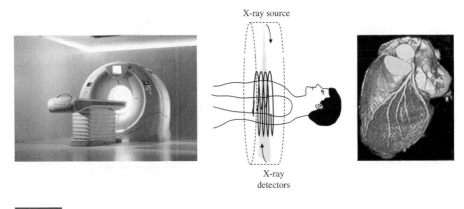

X-ray source

X-ray
detectors

Figure 2.2

(left) A modern helical CT scanner. (centre) The X-ray tube and bank of detectors (typically several hundred, aligned parallel to one another) rotate together while the patient is slowly slid through the beam. The two-dimensional rotational and one-dimensional linear translation together enable a full three-dimensional data set to be acquired very rapidly. (right) An example of a surface rendering of a three-dimensional CT data set of the human heart, showing the coronary arteries on the exterior.

the coronary arteries. The only disadvantage of a CT scan compared to a planar X-ray is the much higher radiation dose.

2.2   The X-ray tube

For both planar radiography and CT the X-ray source is a specialized piece of equipment known as an X-ray tube. A photograph of an X-ray tube and a schematic diagram of its major components are shown in Figure 2.3. All of the components of the X-ray system are contained within an evacuated vessel. The evacuated vessel is surrounded by oil for both cooling and electrical isolation. The whole assembly is surrounded by a lead shield with a glass window, through which the X-ray beam is emitted.

X-rays are produced by a beam of high energy electrons striking the surface of a metal target. A negatively-charged cathode acts as the source of these electrons, and consists of a small helix of thin tungsten wire, through which an electric current is passed. When the temperature of the wire reaches ~2200 °C, electrons have sufficient energy to leave the metal surface. In order to produce a tight beam of electrons, a negatively-charged 'focusing cup' surrounds the cathode. A large positive voltage is applied to a metal target, which thus forms an anode. A potential difference between the anode and cathode of between 25 and 140 kV (depending upon the particular type of clinical study) is applied, such that the electrons produced at the cathode are attracted to the anode, striking it at

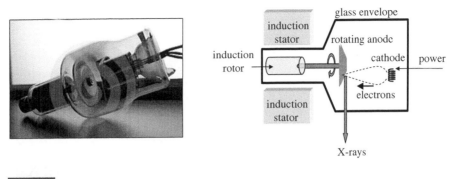

Figure 2.3

(left) An X-ray tube enclosed in an evacuated glass enclosure. (right) The individual components of an X-ray tube.

high velocities. This potential difference is known as the accelerating voltage, or kVp.

When the high energy electrons strike the anode surface, part of their kinetic energy is converted into X-rays by mechanisms covered in detail in Section 2.3. The metal anode must be able to produce X-rays efficiently, and also be able to withstand the very high temperatures generated. In terms of efficiency, the higher the atomic number of the metal in the target, the higher the efficiency of X-ray production. The most commonly used metal is tungsten which has a high atomic number, 74, and a melting point of 3370 °C. In addition it has good thermal conductivity and a low vapour pressure, which allows a strong vacuum to be established within the X-ray tube, thus providing the electrons with an unimpeded path between cathode and anode. Even with the high efficiency of tungsten only ~1% of the energy of the electrons is converted into X-rays: the remainder is dissipated in heat. The tungsten target of the anode is about 0.7 mm thick and forms a cylindrical disk which rotates at high speed, ~3000 rpm, in order to reduce the localized heating. The power for rotation comes from a set of induction rotors and stators, as shown in Figure 2.3. In practice, a tungsten–rhenium (2–10% rhenium) alloy is used for extra mechanical stability of the target. As mentioned earlier, digital mammography requires very low energy X-rays, and for these types of application the metal in the anode is molybdenum rather than tungsten.

In order to produce a narrow beam of electrons, a negatively-charged focusing cup is constructed around the cathode filament. In fact, many X-ray tubes contain two cathode filaments of different length, each with a focusing cup, as shown in Figure 2.4.

In order to achieve a well-defined small area in which the X-rays are created, the anode is bevelled at an angle between 8 and 17°, with 12–15° being the usual

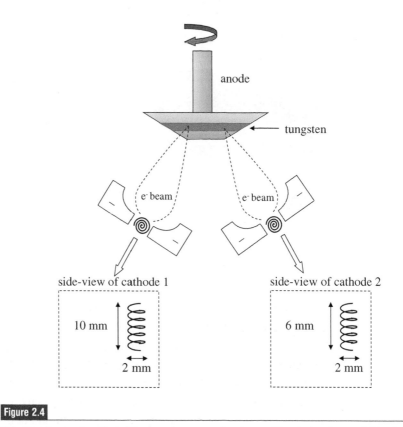

Top view showing the effect of the focusing cup on the shape of the electron beam striking the rotating anode. There are two cathodes (expanded in the side-views) which produce a wider or narrower beam depending upon the particular application. The direction of the X-ray beam produced is out-of-the-page towards the reader.

range. The smaller the angle, the smaller the effective focal spot size (f), shown in Figure 2.5(a), given by:

$$f = F \sin\theta, \tag{2.1}$$

where θ is the bevel angle and F the width of the electron beam. Values of the effective focal spot size range from 0.3 mm for digital mammography to between 0.6 and 1.2 mm for planar radiography and computed tomography. The bevel angle also affects the coverage of the X-ray beam, as shown in Figure 2.5(b), which is given by:

$$\text{Coverage} = 2(\text{source} - \text{patient distance}) \tan\theta. \tag{2.2}$$

In practice, the X-ray beam has a higher intensity at the 'cathode-end' than at the 'anode-end', a phenomenon known as the Heel effect. This effect is due to differences in the distances that X-rays have to travel through the target itself. This

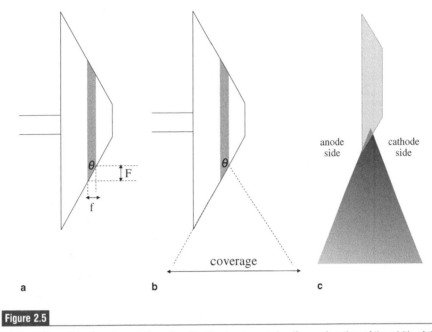

anode side   cathode side

a   b   c

coverage

Figure 2.5

(a) The effect of the bevel angle θ on the effective focal spot size (f) as a function of the width of the electron beam (F). (b) Corresponding diagram for the effect of θ on the coverage of the X-ray beam. (c) Illustration of the Heel effect, in which the X-ray intensity is higher on the 'cathode side' of the beam than on the 'anode side', since the X-rays on the anode side have to travel further through the anode itself before leaving the tube, and are therefore more highly attenuated.

distance is longer for X-rays produced at the anode-side of the target than at the cathode-side, as shown in Figure 2.5 (c), and results in greater absorption of X-rays within the target itself. This means that the signal intensity on one side of a planar radiograph is different from that on the other. Although image processing algorithms can be used to correct for this phenomenon, in practice it is not significantly detrimental to the diagnostic quality of the images.

There are three parameters that can be chosen by the operator for X-ray imaging: the accelerating voltage (kVp), the tube current (mA), and the exposure time. The current that passes from the cathode to the anode is typically between 50 and 400 mA for planar radiography, and up to 1000 mA for CT. The value of the kVp varies from ~25 kV for digital mammography to ~140 kV for bone and chest applications. Physical limitations for the values of kVp and tube current are set by the power rating of the particular X-ray tube, defined as the maximum power dissipated in an exposure time of 0.1 s. For example, a tube with a power rating of 10 kW can operate at a kVp of 125 kV with a tube current of 1 A for ~78 ms. The ability of the X-ray source to achieve a high tube output is ultimately limited by anode heating. The heat generated in the anode is transferred to the tube housing and from there to the insulating oil surrounding the housing. Further heat removal can be achieved by continuously pumping oil or cooling water within the housing.

2.3   The X-ray energy spectrum

X-ray tubes produce X-rays with a wide range of energies, up to a maximum value given by the kVp, as shown in Figure 2.6. The spectrum represents a plot of the relative number of X-rays produced as a function of their energy. When one refers to the energy of the X-ray beam, this number represents the weighted average of all of the different energies, and is typically about two-thirds of the kVp value.

There are two separate mechanisms by which X-rays are produced, one which results in a broad spread of energies, and the other which produces distinct sharp lines, both of which are evident in Figure 2.6. The first mechanism involves an electron passing close to the nucleus of an atom of the metal forming the anode, and being deflected from its original trajectory by the attractive forces from the positively charged nucleus. This deflection results in a loss of electron kinetic energy, and this energy loss is converted into an X-ray. The maximum energy that an X-ray can have corresponds to the entire kinetic energy of the electron

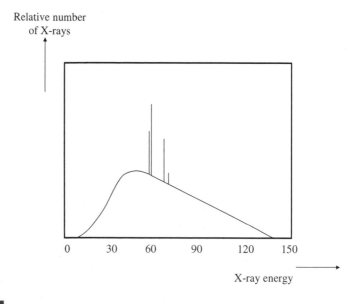

Figure 2.6

The energy spectrum of a beam emitted from an X-ray tube with a tungsten anode operating at 140 kVp. The very low energies are absorbed by the tube itself. Characteristic lines are seen as sharp lines, superimposed upon a broad energy distribution from general radiation.

being transferred to the X-ray, i.e. the kVp value. Given the small size of the nucleus in relation to the entire atom, it is much more likely that the electron will undergo only a partial loss of energy, and so a wide spectrum of X-ray energies is produced: this is termed general radiation or bremsstrahlung (braking radiation in German). Although the distribution decreases roughly linearly with energy, many of the very low energy X-rays are absorbed by the housing of the X-ray tube itself, as evident on the left-hand-side of Figure 2.6.

Sharp peaks are also present in the X-ray energy spectrum, and the energy at which these peaks occur is characteristic of the particular metal used in the anode, hence the name 'characteristic radiation'. If an electron accelerated from the cathode collides with a tightly bound K-shell electron in the anode, this bound electron is ejected and the resulting 'hole' in the K-shell is filled by an electron from an outer (L or M) shell, see Figure 2.7. The difference in binding energies between the electrons in the inner and outer shells is emitted as a single X-ray with a specific energy.

As outlined earlier, the two most commonly-used metals for anodes are tungsten and molybdenum. For tungsten, the K-shell electrons have a binding energy of 69.5 keV. The L-shell has electrons with binding energies between 10.2 and 12.1 keV, and the M-shell between 1.9 and 2.8 keV. Therefore, a characteristic X-ray from an L-to-K electron transition has an energy of ~59 keV, and from an M-to-K transition an energy of ~67 keV: these represent the sharp peaks shown in Figure 2.6. For a molybdenum target, the binding energies of electrons in the K-, L- and M-shells are 20, 2.5–2.8 and 0.4–0.5 keV, respectively. The

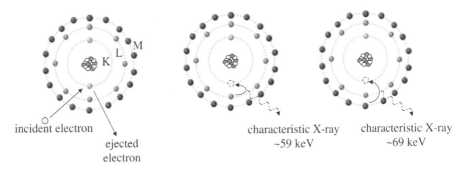

incident electron

ejected electron

characteristic X-ray ~59 keV

characteristic X-ray ~69 keV

Figure 2.7

The chain-of-events involved in production of characteristic radiation from the metal anode in an X-ray tube. (left) A high energy electron from the cathode ejects an inner electron from the metal target in the anode. An outer electron fills the hole in the inner shell and the difference in binding energies of the inner and outer shell electrons is converted into a characteristic X-ray which is emitted. The outer electron can come from the L-shell (centre) or M-shell (right), resulting in two different characteristic X-ray energies.

corresponding energy spectrum is shown in Section 2.10.2 when digital mammography is discussed.

2.4   Interactions of X-rays with the body

In order to produce images with high SNR and high CNR, three basic criteria should be satisfied: (i) sufficient X-rays must be transmitted through the body for a high SNR, (ii) X-ray absorption must be sufficiently different between different tissue-types in order to produce high contrast, and (iii) there must be a method for removing X-rays which are scattered through unknown angles as they pass through the body. For the energies used in diagnostic X-ray imaging, there are two major mechanisms by which X-rays interact with tissue. The first mechanism is the photoelectric interaction with differential attenuation between, in particular, bone and soft tissue. The second mechanism, Compton scattering, involves the X-ray being deflected from its original trajectory. The X-ray energy is reduced, but the scattered X-ray may still have enough energy to reach the detector. Compton scattered X-rays give a random background signal, and so their contribution to the image should be minimized to improve the CNR. There are other mechanisms by which X-rays interact with tissue (such as coherent scattering), but for the energies used in clinical radiography the contributions from these are minor and so are not considered here.

2.4.1   Photoelectric attenuation

The first mechanism, in which tissue *absorbs* X-rays, provides the contrast in X-ray images. These 'photoelectric interactions' are very similar to the phenomenon of characteristic radiation, described in Section 2.3. The first step is that the energy of the incident X-ray is absorbed by tissue, with a tightly bound electron being emitted from either the K- or L-shell, as shown in Figure 2.8. This ejected electron has an energy equal to the difference between the energy of the incident X-ray and the binding energy of the electron. The second step is that an electron from a higher energy level fills the 'hole' with the emission of a 'characteristic' X-ray, with an energy equal to the difference in the binding energies of the two electrons. This characteristic X-ray has a very low energy, a few keV at most, and is absorbed by the tissue. The net result of the photoelectric effect in tissue, therefore, is that the incident X-ray is completely absorbed and does not reach the detector. Note that the electronic configurations of the most important elements in tissue, in terms of photoelectric interactions, are: carbon (K2, L4), oxygen (K2, L6) and calcium (K2, L8, M8, N2).

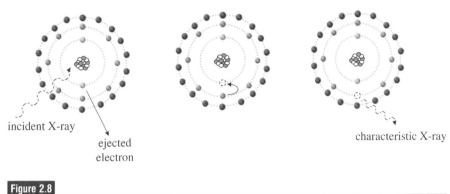

incident X-ray

ejected
electron

characteristic X-ray

Figure 2.8

A photoelectric interaction between an incident X-ray and tissue involves an inner electron being emitted (left), an electron from an outer shell filling the hole in the inner shell (middle), and the difference in the binding energies being transferred to a characteristic X-ray. This X-ray has very low energy and is absorbed after travelling ~1 mm in tissue.

The probability of a photoelectric interaction (P_{pe}) occurring depends on the energy (E) of the incident X-ray, the effective atomic number (Z_{eff}) of the tissue, and the tissue density (ρ):

$$P_{pe} \propto \rho \frac{Z_{eff}^3}{E^3}. \qquad (2.3)$$

The effective atomic number of tissue is ~7.4, of lipid ~6.9, and of bone ~13.8 (the high value is due primarily to the presence of calcium). The relative densities are 1: 0.9: 1.85. Equation (2.3) indicates that, at low X-ray energies, the photoelectric effect produces high constrast between bone (high attenuation) and soft tissue (low attenuation), but that the contrast decreases with increasing X-ray energy. This is further expanded upon in Section 2.5.

2.4.2 Compton scattering

Compton scattering refers to the interaction between an incident X-ray and a loosely bound electron in an outer shell of an atom in tissue. In Compton scattering a small fraction of the incident X-ray energy is transferred to this loosely-bound electron. With the additional energy, the electron is ejected, and the X-ray is deflected from its original path by an angle θ, as shown in Figure 2.9.

The energy of the scattered X-ray can be calculated by applying the laws of conservation of momentum and energy. The standard Compton equation computes the change in wavelength between the incident and scattered X-ray, which is given by:

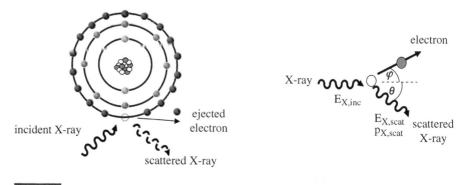

Figure 2.9

Compton scattering of an incident X-ray involves an outer electron being ejected from a tissue molecule (left), with the X-ray being scattered at an angle θ with respect to its initial trajectory (right).

$$\Delta\lambda = \frac{h}{m_0 c}(1 - \cos\theta), \qquad (2.4)$$

where m_0 is the rest mass of the ejected electron, and c is the speed of light. This change in wavelength can easily be converted into the relevant loss in energy (ΔE):

$$\Delta E = E_{X,inc} - E_{X,scat} = \frac{hc}{\lambda_{inc}} - \frac{hc}{\lambda_{scat}}. \qquad (2.5)$$

The energy of the scattered X-ray is then given by:

$$E_{X,scat} = \frac{E_{X,inc}}{1 + \left(\frac{E_{X,inc}}{mc^2}\right)(1 - \cos\theta)}. \qquad (2.6)$$

Figure 2.10 shows a graph of scattered X-ray energy vs. scatter angle for an incident energy of 70 keV. As can be seen from the graph, the energy of the X-ray is reduced only by a very small amount even for quite large deflection angles, and so it is very likely that it will pass through the body and be detected as if it were primary radiation, i.e. radiation which has not been scattered at all. Of course, if the scatter angle is very large the trajectory of the scattered X-ray will miss the detector, and the X-ray will effectively have been attenuated.

The probability of an X-ray undergoing Compton scattering is, to first order, independent of atomic number, is proportional to the tissue electron density, and is only weakly dependent on the energy of the incident X-ray.

At low X-ray energies, the photoelectric effect dominates over Compton scattering. Since the Z_{eff} of bone is approximately twice that of tissue, there is far greater attenuation in bone than in tissue, and excellent tissue contrast. However, at higher X-ray energies the contribution from Compton scattering becomes

Scatter angle (degrees)

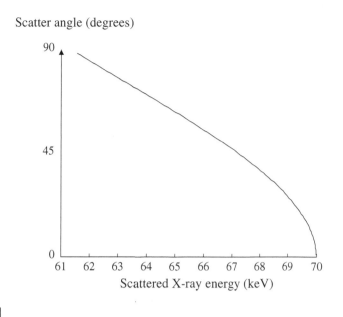

Scattered X-ray energy (keV)

The energy of a Compton-scattered X-ray as a function of the scatter angle for a 70 keV incident energy.

more important, and contrast therefore drops, as described in detail in the next section.

2.5 X-ray linear and mass attenuation coefficients

The attenuation of X-rays through the body has been experimentally determined to be an exponential process with respect to distance travelled. The exponential function can be characterized in terms of a tissue linear attenuation coefficient (μ). The value of μ depends upon the energy of the incident X-rays. One can therefore express the number (N) of X-rays transmitted through a certain thickness (x) of tissue as:

$$N = N_0 e^{-\mu(E)x}, \tag{2.7}$$

where N_o is of the number of incident X-rays. The value of μ is the sum of the individual contributions from photoelectric absorption and Compton scattering:

$$\mu(E) = \mu(E)_{photoelectric} + \mu(E)_{Compton}. \tag{2.8}$$

X-ray attenuation in tissue is most often characterized in terms of a mass attenuation coefficient (μ/ρ), measured in units of $cm^2 g^{-1}$. Figure 2.11 shows

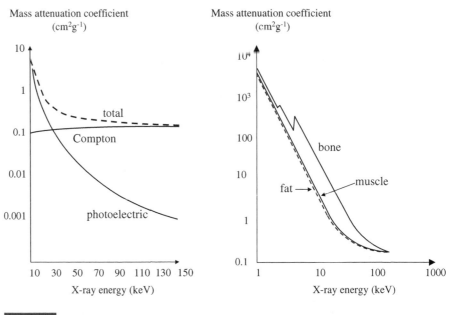

Figure 2.11

(left) The individual contributions from photoelectric attenuation and Compton scatter add together to give a net tissue linear attenuation coefficient (the specific data are shown for water). The contribution from the photoelectric effect dominates at low X-ray energies, but Compton scatter is the more important term at high energies. (right) The mass attenuation coefficient of lipid, muscle and bone as a function of X-ray energy.

the relative contributions of photoelectric and Compton interactions as a function of the incident X-ray energy. As outlined earlier, the contribution from photoelectric interactions dominates at lower energies, whereas Compton scattering is more important at higher energies.

Figure 2.11 also shows the mass attenuation coefficients of bone, soft tissue and lipid as a function of the incident X-ray energy. At low incident X-ray energies bone has by far the highest mass attenuation coefficient, due to the prevalence of photoelectric interactions and the high effective atomic number of bone (13.8) compared to tissue (7.4) and lipid (6.9). As the X-ray energy increases, the values of the mass attenuation coefficient become much lower for all tissues. At X-ray energies greater than about 80 keV, the difference in the mass attenuation coefficients of bone and soft-tissue is less than a factor of 2. There is also relatively little difference between the attenuation coefficients for soft tissue and fat due to their closeness in effective atomic number.

An important feature in Figure 2.11 is the sharp discontinuities in the absorption coefficient of bone at two distinct energies. This phenomenon is known as a K-edge: at an energy just higher than the K-shell binding energy of the particular atom (calcium for bone), the probability of photoelectric interactions increases dramatically, typically by a factor of 5 to 8. One can see that, without these jumps, the attenuation of bone would be very similar to that of muscle and lipid. The phenomenon of a K-edge is also critical in the design of both X-ray contrast agents and X-ray detectors, which are covered later in this chapter.

The attenuation properties of tissue can also be described in terms of the half-value layer (HVL), which as the name suggests is the thickness of tissue which reduces the intensity of the X-ray beam by a factor of one-half. From Equation (2.7), the value of the HVL is given by $(\ln 2)/\mu$. At an X-ray energy of 100 keV, for example, the HVL for muscle is 3.9 cm and for bone is 2.3 cm: the corresponding numbers at 30 keV (relevant for mammography) are 1.8 cm and 0.4 cm, respectively.

Example 2.1 If the thickness of the chest is 20 cm, what percentage of X-rays are transmitted through the chest at an incident X-ray energy of 70 keV assuming HVL values of 3.5 and 1.8 cm^{-1} for muscle and bone, respectively, and the bone thickness to be 4 cm and the tissue thickness 16 cm?

Solution For the muscle, the value of μ is given by $(\ln 2)/3.5{\sim}0.2$ cm^{-1}. For 16 cm of tissue:

$$\frac{N}{N_0} = e^{-(0.2)16} = 0.04.$$

For bone the value of μ is $(\ln 2)/1.8{\sim}0.4$ cm^{-1}. For 4 cm of bone:

$$\frac{N}{N_0} = e^{-(0.4)4} = 0.2.$$

Therefore, overall the percentage is given by $100 \times (0.2 \times 0.04) = 0.8\%$.

2.6 Instrumentation for planar radiography

In addition to the X-ray tube, the other basic components of a planar X-ray radiography system are: (i) a collimator to reduce the patient dose and amount of Compton scattered X-rays, (ii) an anti-scatter grid to reduce further the contribution of scattered X-rays to the image, and (iii) a digital detector which converts the energy of the transmitted X-rays into light: the light is then converted into a voltage using photodiodes, and this voltage is digitized using an analogue-to-digital converter, as covered in Chapter 1.

2.6.1 Collimators

The coverage of the X-ray beam from the X-ray tube is determined by the bevel angle of the anode in the X-ray tube, as shown in Section 2.2. By the time the beam reaches the patient, the beam can be much wider than the field-of-view (FOV) which is being imaged. This has two undesirable effects, the first of which is that the patient dose is unnecessarily high. The second effect is that the number of Compton scattered X-rays contributing to the image is also unnecessarily increased, since X-rays interact with tissue outside the FOV, and are scattered and detected. In order to restrict the dimensions of the beam to the imaging FOV a collimator (also called a beam-restrictor) is placed between the X-ray source and the patient. The collimator consists of sheets of lead, which can be slid over one another to restrict the beam in either one or two dimensions.

2.6.2 Anti-scatter grids

Compton scattered X-rays provide little spatial information, and contribute to a background signal which reduces the image contrast. For example, Figure 2.12 shows X-ray images from a model of the human pelvis. The areas around the 'bones' in the model should be black in the images since they contain only air. However, in regions close to the bone, these areas show up with a high signal intensity due to Compton scatter.

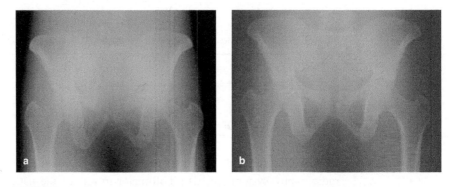

Figure 2.12

Images showing the effects of an anti-scatter grid on the CNR of a planar X-ray image. The images are produced from a pelvic phantom, which simulates the absorption properties of the human pelvis. (a) No anti-scatter grid: there is a large background signal from Compton-scattered X-rays which reduces the CNR of the image. (b) With an anti-scatter grid in place the overall signal intensity of the image is reduced, but the CNR is improved significantly.

To reduce the contribution from secondary radiation, an anti-scatter grid is placed between the patient and the X-ray detector. Certain manufacturers incorporate this grid into the detector itself, for example in computed radiography covered in Section 2.7.1. This grid consists of parallel strips of lead foil with aluminium used as a spacer between the strips, as shown in Figure 2.13. Since the X-ray beam is in fact slightly diverging, as shown in Figure 2.5 (b), the anti-scatter grid can also be manufactured at the same diverging angle with a focal point ~180 cm from the grid. The degree to which the contribution from Compton scattering is reduced is dictated by the thickness (t), length (h) and separation (d) of the lead strips. The grid is characterized by two properties, the grid ratio and grid frequency given by:

$$\text{grid ratio} = \frac{h}{d} \quad \text{grid frequency} = \frac{1}{d + t}. \tag{2.9}$$

Typical values of the grid ratio range from 4:1 to 16:1 and grid frequency from 5–7 lines mm^{-1}. The improvement in image contrast does, however, come at a cost in terms of an increase in the X-ray dose which is required to produce a given image intensity while using an anti-scatter grid. Having finite thickness, the lead septa absorb some primary radiation, and X-rays which are scattered only at very small angles (and therefore contain useful spatial information) are also absorbed. This trade-off can be characterized using a parameter known as the Bucky factor

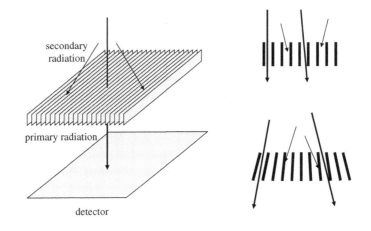

secondary radiation

primary radiation

detector

Figure 2.13

(left) Basic design of an anti-scatter grid, with thin lead septa aligned in either a parallel (top right) or slightly diverging (bottom right) geometry. The thick arrows show primary radiation which passes through the anti-scatter grid, and the thin arrows correspond to secondary Compton-scattered radiation which is stopped by the grid.

(BF). If an equal X-ray dose is incident upon the detector in the presence and absence of an anti-scatter grid, then the dose that is delivered to the patient increases by a factor BF. Typical values of BF are between 4 and 10. In Figure 2.12(b), for example, the image contrast is improved significantly by use of an anti-scatter grid: however, the X-ray dose to the patient is almost ten times higher than for the image in Figure 2.12(a) acquired without an anti-scatter grid.

2.7   X-ray detectors

Traditional X-ray film is essentially a thing of the past, with current diagnoses being performed almost exclusively from digital images displayed on high resolution computer screens. In addition to the higher quality images made possible using digital detectors, the ability to store and transfer images easily through large medical data centres via so-called picture archiving and communication systems (PACS) has become extremely important. There are two basic digital detector technologies which are currently used, computed radiography and digital radiography. The former is currently cheaper and more widespread, but is anticipated to be superseded by the latter technology within the next decade, especially as the costs of digital radiography fall.

2.7.1   Computed radiography

Computed radiography (CR) instrumentation consists of a detector plate and a CR reader which digitizes the plate after the X-ray image has been acquired. The CR plate consists of a thin layer of phosphor crystals, most commonly barium fluorohalide activated with europium ions ($BaFX:Eu^{2+}$), where the halide X is a mixture of bromine and iodine. The plate size ranges from 18×24 cm for mammography to 35×43 cm for chest radiography. The plates can be categorized as either high resolution (HR), usually used for mammography, or standard for general applications. Note that HR plates have a thinner phosphor layer (~140 μm) compared to standard plates (230 μm), and the phosphor crystals are physically smaller [1].

The CR plates convert the X-rays which pass through the patient and the anti-scatter grid into light. When X-rays strike the plate they release electrons in the phosphor layer: these electrons are trapped for a timescale of hours in sites formed by dislocations in the phosphor crystal lattice. This effectively forms a 'latent' image, i.e. one which is present but is not immediately visible. The CR plate is protected by a light-tight cassette which is transparent to X-rays. After the image has been acquired, the cassette is fed into a CR reader. There are many types of reader, one of the more advanced being a line-scan readout CR, a schematic of which is shown in Figure 2.14. A linear array of many laser-diodes and small focusing lenses is used, illuminating an area of ~50 μm diameter for each laser-diode/lens combination. The laser causes most of the trapped electrons in the phosphor to return to the ground state, and as they do they emit the difference in energy between excited and ground states as light at the blue end of the spectrum. This light is detected using an array of small lenses and photodiodes which are sensitive to blue light. The photodiodes convert light into a voltage, and the output voltage from each photodiode is amplified, filtered and digitized. An entire plate can be read and digitized in ~10 seconds. After it has been read, the plate is then 'bleached' using several high-intensity lights, and inserted into a fresh cassette to be reused.

There are many variations on the basic CR plate. As can be appreciated from Figure 2.14, up to one-half of the light produced by the laser diodes may not be recorded, since it can escape through the bottom of the detector. For a standard CR plate, the base for the phosphor crystals is made of a reflective layer, which improves the detection efficiency. However, it reduces the spatial resolution since the path that reflected light has to travel before being detected is twice as long, and the light spreads out as it travels (referred to as a broadened light spread function). For applications such as digital mammography, which requires very high resolution, an absorbent layer is placed at the bottom of the detector to reduce the light spread function to a minimum: however, this also results in reduced efficiency. A more sophisticated way to capture a higher percentage of the light is to use a dual-sided CR plate, in which there are phosphor layers on both sides of a transparent plastic base, but this requires a more sophisticated CR reader.

New materials are also being used in CR plates. An example is $CsBr:Eu^{2+}$, which has a structure of thin columnar crystals which are aligned perpendicular to the surface of the plate. These effectively act as very thin optical fibres,

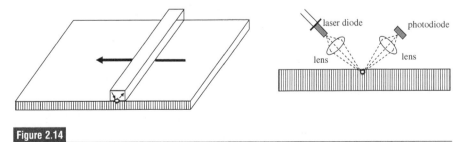

Figure 2.14

A computed radiography reader. The reader consists of a large array of laser diodes and photodiodes, and this array is rapidly moved from right-to-left across the plate to produce the entire image.

preventing light from spreading through the plate (thus reducing the light spread function), and so have a higher intrinsic spatial resolution than $BaFX:Eu^{2+}$ crystals, which are randomly oriented. The regular crystal structure of $CsBr:Eu^{2+}$ also results in a much higher packing efficiency, i.e. a greater number of crystals per unit area, which increases the sensivity compared to $BaFX:Eu^{2+}$. Using $CsBr:Eu^{2+}$ allows the thickness of the phosphor layer to be increased to 600 µm, further increasing the number of X-rays that are absorbed.

The dynamic range of a CR system is very high: typically the signal output is linear with respect to the X-ray input dose over a range of four orders-of-magnitude. The spatial resolution is limited by the size of the laser beam used in signal readout, the number of data points which are sampled, and the degree of scatter of the laser beam by the crystals in the phosphor screen. Note that HR plates have smaller and thinner crystals, and therefore higher spatial resolution. Pixels are sampled every 50 µm, and CR plates are digitized as 4096×4096 (HR) or 2048×2048 matrix sizes (standard). The SNR of a standard image plate is roughly twice that of a HR plate for the same input dose. Using a dual-sided CR plate increases the SNR by close to a factor of 2 compared to single-sided, and using new $CsBr:Eu^{2+}$ based plates increases the SNR by an additional factor of 2.

2.7.2 Digital radiography

There are two types of digital radiography (DR) detectors, indirect- and direct-conversion. Indirect-conversion is most commonly used, the term 'indirect' referring to the fact that X-ray energy is first converted into light by a CsI:Tl scintillator, and then the light is converted into a voltage using a two-dimensional array of photodiodes. Caesium and iodine have K-edges at 36 and 33.2 keV, with high atomic numbers of 55 and 53, respectively: therefore, the X-ray attenuation coefficient of CsI is very high, as shown in Figure 2.15, making it a highly efficient detector.

A schematic of an indirect-conversion DR detector is shown in Figure 2.16. The CsI layer consists of many thin, rod-shaped, CsI:Tl 'needle crystals' (approximately 5 µm in diameter) aligned parallel to one another and extending from the top surface of the CsI layer to the substrate on which they are manufactured. The needle structure gives excellent packing efficiency ($>80\%$) to enhance X-ray absorption and, similarly to CR, it also channels light effectively, preventing it from spreading and blurring the image. For planar radiography the thickness of the CsI:Tl layer is ~0.6 mm.

The large flat-panel detector (FPD), which lies directly underneath the CsI:Tl layer consists of thin-film transistor (TFT) arrays, the same technology as is used in

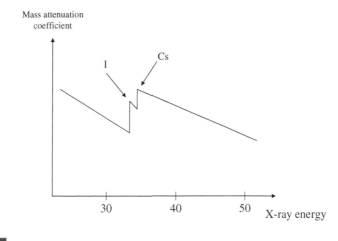

Mass attenuation coefficient

I

Cs

30   40   50   X-ray energy

Figure 2.15

The attenuation coefficient of CsI:Tl as a function of the incident X-ray energy. Each of the elements has a K-edge which increases absorption significantly.

computer screens [2]. Unlike CR, DR does not need a separate read-out device. The FPD is fabricated on a glass substrate. Then a thin-film amorphous silicon transistor array is layered on to the glass. Amorphous silicon is used rather than the crystalline form which is used in microchip fabrication, since it has the advantage that it can be repeatedly exposed to high intensity X-rays without damage. Each pixel of the detector consists of a fabricated photodiode, storage capacitor and TFT switch.

When an X-ray is absorbed in a CsI rod, the CsI scintillates and produces light in the green part of the spectrum. The light undergoes internal reflection within the fibre and is emitted from one end of the fibre on to the TFT array. The light is converted to an electrical signal by the photodiodes in the TFT array and stored in capacitors which are formed at the junction of the photodiodes. This signal is then read out line-by-line in parallel using a multiplexer. The signals are amplified and digitized using a 14-bit analogue-to-digital (A/D) converter.

A typical commercial DR system has flat-panel dimensions of 43×43 cm, with a TFT array of 3001×3001 elements corresponding to a pixel sampling interval of 143 μm. An anti-scatter grid with a grid ratio of ~13:1 and a strip line density of ~70 lines per cm is used for scatter rejection. It is packaged into a device approximately 50×50 cm square, 4.5 cm thick, with a weight of ~20 kilogrammes.

The alternative form of DR detection using direct conversion, as the name suggests, eliminates the intermediate step of converting X-ray energy into light, and uses direct absorption of the X-ray photons to produce an electrical signal. Materials such as amorphous selenium (alloyed with arsenic to prevent recrystallization) have been used, although with an atomic number of 34 and K-edge

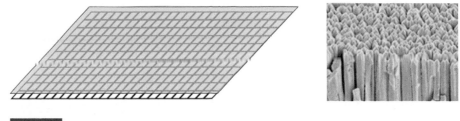

(left) A thin CsI:Tl layer (shaded) placed on top of a SiH active matrix array. (right) An electron micrograph showing the needle-like structure of the crystals of CsI:Tl.

at 13 keV, X-ray absorption is not as efficient as for CsI:Tl. The amorphous selenium material is layered on top of an amorphous Si-H array, as described previously. Many new materials are being investigated for direct conversion radiography, but currently the properties of the indirect-conversion detectors are more favourable.

2.8   Quantitative characteristics of planar X-ray images

As outlined in Chapter 1, the three most common quantitative parameters used to measure the 'quality' of an image are the SNR, spatial resolution and CNR. An image ideally has a high value of each of these parameters, but there are usually instrumental and operational trade-offs.

2.8.1   Signal-to-noise

Ideally, with no patient present, the number of X-rays striking each part of the detector would be exactly the same. However, there are slight variations in the number of photons per square millimetre, for example, around a mean value. This variation introduces a statistical fluctuation into the signal intensity of each pixel, which is represented as noise in the image. If the number of X-rays produced per unit area is plotted, one gets a Poisson distribution, shown in Figure 2.17.

The distribution looks similar to the more familiar Normal distribution (from basic statistics), but is described by a different mathematical function. The probability, P(N), that N X-rays strike the detector plate per unit area is given by:

$$P(N) = \frac{\mu^{N}e^{-\mu}}{N!}, \tag{2.10}$$

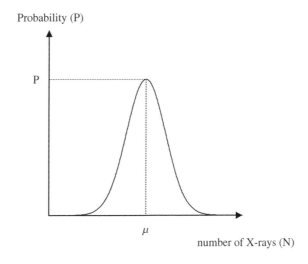

Figure 2.17

The probability of a certain number of X-rays striking a unit area of the detector. The statistical uncertainty in this number is represented by the standard deviation (σ) of the Poisson distribution.

where μ is the mean value. For the Poisson distribution the value of σ is given by:

$$\sigma = \sqrt{\mu}. \tag{2.11}$$

Figure 2.18 shows three plots of P(N) vs N for increasing values of N. For very large values of N, the graph approaches a delta function, and therefore the value of μ approaches that of N. The SNR, defined in Chapter 1 as the ratio of the signal to the standard deviation of the noise, is therefore given by N/σ, or:

$$\text{SNR} \propto \sqrt{N}. \tag{2.12}$$

Doubling the image SNR, therefore, requires four times the number of X-rays to be detected, increasing the radiation dose also by a factor of 4.

Given the relationship between the SNR and number of X-rays detected, operational factors that affect the SNR include:

(i) *the tube current and exposure time*: the SNR is proportional to the square root of the product of these two quantities,

(ii) *the tube kVp*: the higher the kVp value the greater the tissue penetration of the higher energy X-rays, and so the higher the SNR: this is a non-linear effect,

(iii) *the patient size and part of the body being imaged:* the greater the thickness of tissue through which the X-rays have to travel, and the higher the X-ray attenuation due to bone, the lower the SNR,

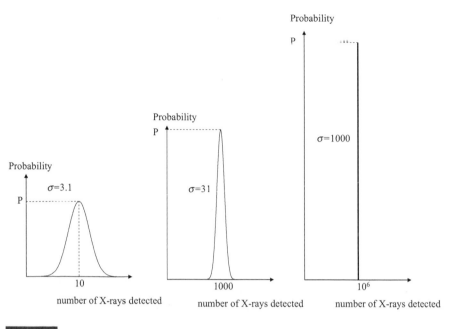

Figure 2.18

Plots of a Poisson distribution with increasing number of X-rays produced. As the number increases, the distribution becomes narrower, with the mean number of events and the total number of events converging to the same value.

(iv) *the geometry of the anti-scatter grid*: an anti-scatter grid with a large grid ratio attenuates a greater degree of Compton scattered X-rays than one with a smaller ratio, and therefore reduces the image SNR (but improves the CNR),

(v) *the efficiency of the detector*: this can be quantified using a parameter known as the detector quantum efficiency (DQE), defined as:

$$DQE = \left[\frac{SNR_{out}}{SNR_{in}}\right]^2, \qquad (2.13)$$

where the subscripts 'in' and 'out' refer to the input SNR to, and output SNR from, the detector. The value of the DQE is always less than 1, since the detector must introduce some noise into the system, but the higher the DQE the higher the SNR for a given number of X-rays entering the detector. For example, the DQE of a standard CR plate has a value ~0.25, for a high resolution CR plate the DQE is ~0.12. Using a dual-sided read CR increases the DQE to ~0.4. The highest DQE ~0.8 is for $CsBr:Eu^{2+}$ based plates.

As mentioned previously, if a CR or DR plate is exposed to an X-ray beam with no patient present, then the image intensity should be absolutely uniform.

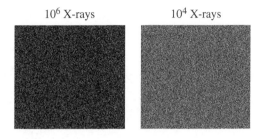

Figure 2.19

The effect of radiation dose (total number of incident X-rays) on the SNR of a planar image with no patient in place. The image on the left has 100 times the number of X-rays per pixel, and so has 10 times higher SNR.

However, even assuming a perfect detector response, there are still small variations in the image intensity over the plate, as shown in Figure 2.19.

2.8.2 Spatial resolution

As discussed in Chapter 1, the overall spatial resolution is a combination of the contributions from each part of the imaging process. For planar radiography, the major contributions are:

(i) The size of the effective X-ray focal spot and the relative distances between the X-ray tube and the patient, and the X-ray tube and the detector. The finite size of the effective focal spot of the X-ray tube results in 'geometric unsharpness' of the image, as shown in Figure 2.20. The size of the 'penumbra' region, denoted P, is given by:

$$P = \frac{f(S_1 - S_0)}{S_0}.\qquad(2.14)$$

To improve the image spatial resolution, therefore, the value of S_0 should be as large, and the value of f as small, as possible, with the patient placed directly on top of the detector.

(ii) The properties of the X-ray detector. As outlined in Section 2.7, the spatial resolution depends upon the exact physical make-up of the phosphor layer of the detector, whether it is single- or double-sided, and the number of pixels in the image.

As covered in Chapter 1, the overall MTF is given by the convolution of the individual MTFs from each component of the imaging system. In order to estimate

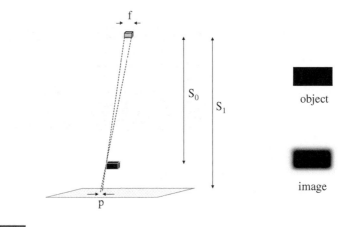

f

S_0

S_1

object

image

p

A finite effective spot size as well as the tube–patient (S_0) and tube–detector (S_1) distances determine the spatial resolution of the image. The 'geometric unsharpness' or penumbra (P) causes features and edges in the image to become blurred, as shown on the right.

these values, the most useful measure of spatial resolution for X-radiography is the line spread function (LSF), which is measured using a grid consisting of parallel lead septa.

2.8.3 Contrast-to-noise

The CNR depends upon three different types of factor: the first determines the relative contribution of Compton-scattered X-rays (which reduce the CNR), the second affects the SNR (covered in Section 2.8.1), and the third contributes to the spatial resolution (covered in Section 2.8.2).

Factors affecting the contribution of Compton-scattered X-rays include:

(i) *The X-ray energy spectrum.* For low kVp values, the photoelectric effect dominates, and the values of μ_{bone} and μ_{tissue}, for example, are substantially different. If high energy X-rays are used, then Compton scattering is the predominant interaction, and the contrast is reduced considerably. However, the dose of low-energy X-rays must be much greater than that of high-energy X-rays for a given image SNR,

(ii) *The field-of-view (FOV) of the X-ray image* – for values of the FOV between approximately 10 and 30 cm, the proportion of Compton scattered radiation reaching the detector increases linearly with the FOV, and therefore the CNR is reduced with increasing FOV. Above a FOV of 30 cm, the proportion remains constant,

(iii) *The thickness of the body part being imaged* – the thicker the section, then the larger the contribution from Compton scattered X-rays and the lower the number of X-rays detected. Both factors reduce the CNR of the image,

(iv) *The geometry of the anti-scatter grid* – as outlined in Section 2.8.1, there is a trade-off between the SNR of the image and the contribution of Compton scattered X-rays to the image.

2.9 X-ray contrast agents

In medical imaging the term 'contrast agent' refers to a chemical substance which is introduced into the body (either orally or injected into the bloodstream). The substance accumulates, either passively or via active transport, in a particular organ or structure in the body and enhances the contrast between that structure and the surrounding tissue. Contrast agents are often used in X-ray, ultrasound and magnetic resonance imaging: nuclear medicine techniques are by their nature entirely based on injected agents. Contrast agents are designed to give the maximum contrast for the minimum administered dose, and to have as small a degree of adverse side-effects as possible.

X-ray contrast agents are designed to be very efficient at absorbing X-rays, i.e. to have a strong contribution from photoelectric interactions. There are two basic classes of X-ray contrast agent. The first is used for gastrointestinal (GI) tract disorders and is administered orally, rectally or via a nasal cannula: the second is based on water-soluble iodinated compounds which are injected into the bloodstream, and are used to visualize the vasculature in the brain, heart or peripheral arteries and veins.

2.9.1 Contrast agents for the GI tract

The contrast agent barium sulphate is used to investigate abnormalities of the GI tract such as ulcers, polyps, tumours or hernias. Barium has a K-edge at 37.4 keV, and so is a very efficient absorber of X-rays. Barium sulphate is a powder, which is prepared for patient administration as a thick suspension in water. For studies of the upper GI tract, barium sulphate is administered orally. Rectal administration is used for investigations of the lower GI tract. The agent essentially fills the entire lumen and so areas in which it is absent are visible as areas of low X-ray absorption. An example of an adenocarcinoma of the colon is shown in Figure 2.21. As an enema, barium sulphate can also be used as a 'double contrast agent': barium sulphate is administered first, followed by air. The barium sulphate coats the inner

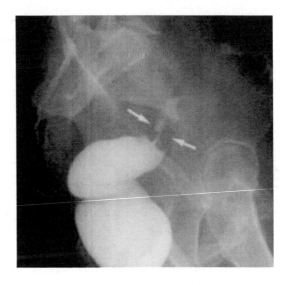

Figure 2.21

A barium sulphate enhanced image of the colon shows an adenocarcinoma (white arrows). The high attenuation of the barium sulphate produces a very high (white) image intensity.

surface of the GI tract and then the air distends the lumen. This double agent approach is used to characterize small pathologies in the large intestine, colon and rectum.

2.9.2   Iodine-based contrast agents

More than 40 million clinical studies are performed every year using iodine-based contrast media, which are administered intravenously into the patient. The reason for choosing iodine is that it has a K-edge at 33.2 keV and so there is substantially increased X-ray attenuation in blood. This allows very small vessels down to ~50 μm diameter to be detected. As with all contrast agents, safety is the major concern, and so the agent must be designed to be as effective as possible at the lowest dose and produce the minimum number of side-effects. All currently-used agents are based on a tri-iodinated benzene ring, with different side-groups (denoted R in Figure 2.22), which dictate the pharmacokinetic properties of the particular agent. A tri-iodinated structure contains the maximum number of iodine atoms, which reduces the required dose. To reduce adverse side-effects the contrast media are non-ionic with low osmolarity. The highest biocompatibility comes from agents such as iodixanol, which have an osmolarity very close to that of blood and CSF (290 mOsm/kg).

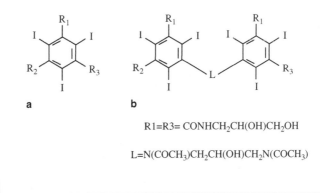

a   b

R1=R3= CONHCH$_2$CH(OH)CH$_2$OH

L=N(COCH$_3$)CH$_2$CH(OH)CH$_2$N(COCH$_3$)

Figure 2.22

(a) Generic formula for a monomeric iodinated X-ray contrast agent. The side-groups R1, R2 and R3 can all be the same or different. (b) Generic form of a dimeric agent, in which the two benzene rings are joined by a chemical linker (L). The chemical structure of iodixanol, which is both iso-osmolar with blood and also non-ionic, is shown.

As shown in Figure 2.22, contrast agents can be monomeric or dimeric. The range of molecular weights of the dimeric agents is 1300–1600, and 650–800 for the monomeric equivalents. The osmolarity of the dimers is much lower than that of the monomers. Each agent contains between 270 and 370 mg of iodine per ml. The agents exhibit very low binding to plasma proteins in the blood, and so are excreted unmetabolized in the urine within 24 hours.

One major use of iodinated contrast agents is digital subtraction angiography, covered in Section 2.10.1. In addition, iodinated X-ray contrast agents are used for intravenous urography, pyelography and cholangiography. In computed tomography, iodinated agents are used in ~50% of scans.

2.10 Specialized X-ray imaging techniques

In addition to planar X-ray imaging, there are a number of different specialized imaging techniques which use X-rays, the main examples of which are described in the following sections.

2.10.1 Digital subtraction angiography

Digital subtraction angiography (DSA) produces very high resolution images of the vasculature in the body, being able to resolve small blood vessels which are less than 100 μm in diameter. The procedure involves acquiring a regular image, then injecting a bolus of iodinated contrast agent into the bloodstream, acquiring a second image, and then performing image subtraction of the two digital images.

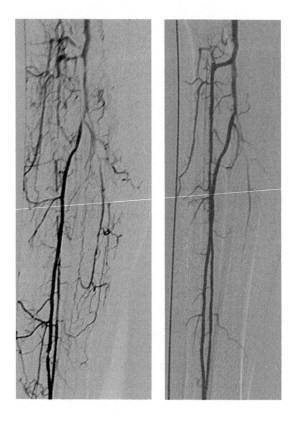

Figure 2.23

Digital subtraction angiograms showing fine vessel structures. The vessels containing iodinated contrast agent are shown as dark areas in the subtraction images.

Examples of DSAs are shown in Figure 2.23. DSA is used to investigate diseases such as stenoses and clotting of arteries and veins, and irregularities in systemic blood flow.

2.10.2 Digital mammography

Digital X-ray mammography is used to detect small tumours or microcalcifications in the breast. Very high spatial resolution and CNR are needed to detect these types of pathology, which can be less than 1 mm in diameter. A low radiation dose is especially important to avoid tissue damage. A specialized X-ray tube is used, with an anode target made from molybdenum (rather than tungsten). Molybdenum has two K-edges at 17.9 and 19.6 keV, as shown in Figure 2.24. The cathode filament is flat, rather than helical, in order to produce a more focused electron beam. The bevel angle of the anode is reduced to produce an effective focal spot size of

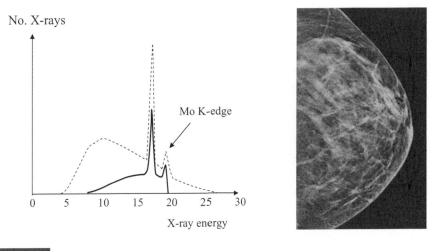

Figure 2.24

(left) The X-ray spectrum used for digital mammography. The kVp of the X-ray tube is 26 keV. The anode is made from molybdenum and produces a substantial number of low energy X-rays (dashed line). A 30 μm thickness molybdenum filter is used to reduce the contribution from very low energy X-rays (solid line). (right) Example of a digital mammogram, showing very high spatial resolution.

0.3 mm or less. The glass window in the X-ray tube is replaced by one fabricated from beryllium to reduce the degree of filtering of the low energy X-rays. A molybdenum filter (30 μm thickness) is used to reduce the amount of high energy X-rays ($>$ 20 keV) which would otherwise give an increased patient dose without improving image quality, as is also shown in Figure 2.24. Occasionally, with a radio-opaque breast, in which attenuation of X-rays is particularly high, an aluminium filter can be used instead of molybdenum.

As described previously, the detector can either be CR or DR-based. The highest spatial resolution configuration is used in either case. To reduce the effects of geometric unsharpness, a large focal-spot-to-detector distance (45 to 80 cm) is used. A 4:1 or 5:1 grid ratio is used for the anti-scatter grid, with septa density typically between 25 and 50 lines per cm, a septal thickness less than 20 μm, and septal height less than 1 mm. Compression of the breast is necessary, normally to about 4 cm thickness, in order to improve X-ray transmission and reduce the contribution from Compton scatter. The digital mammogram on the right of Figure 2.24 shows the very fine detail that can be obtained.

2.10.3 Digital fluoroscopy

Digital fluoroscopy uses continuous X-ray imaging, and can monitor interventional surgery, for example the placement of catheters, guide-wires, stents and

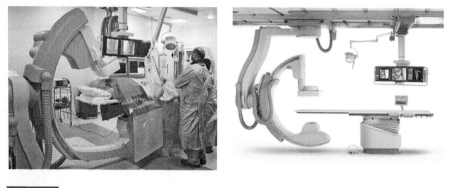

(left) A cardiac catheterization laboratory which uses a digital fluoroscopy unit to monitor placement of stents and pacemakers. (right) A neurointerventional unit, with a C-arm digital fluoroscopy unit.

pacemakers in cardiac catheterization laboratories, as well as for dynamic studies of the GI tract and cardiovascular system using contrast agents. Until very recently, the traditional detector was a digital image intensifier television system (IITV), in which the images produced by an X-ray image intensifier were digitized using a CCD-based device. However, this type of detector is now being replaced by solid-state detectors, which are very similar to indirect-detection digital radiography technology (Section 2.7.2). Some minor modifications to the DR instrumentation are made: for example, the thickness of the CsI:Tl is increased to 550–650 μm to increase the detection efficiency and therefore reduce the required X-ray dose [3]. In recent years most cardiac catheterization laboratories have moved to solid state digital detector technology. An example is shown in Figure 2.25, as well as an example of a neurovascular interventional laboratory.

Solid-state digital fluoroscopy systems use very short pulses of X-rays of ~5–20 ms duration depending upon the type of examination and patient size. Fluoro-scopic images are typically acquired at rates of up to 30 frames per second. The X-ray dose per frame during fluoroscopy can be as low as one one-thousandth of that used during serial image acquisition.

2.11 Clinical applications of planar X-ray imaging

A number of clinical applications of X-ray imaging have already been described. Planar radiography is used for determining the presence and severity of fractures or cracks in the bone structure in the brain, chest, pelvis, arms, legs, hands and feet. Vascular imaging using injected iodine-based contrast agents is performed to study compromised blood-flow, mainly in the brain and heart, but also in the peripheral venous and arterial systems. Diseases of the GI tract can be diagnosed using barium sulphate as a contrast agent, usually with continuous monitoring via X-ray fluoroscopic techniques. Investigations of the urinary tract are among the most common applications of planar X-ray imaging, and are carried out in the form of kidney, ureter and bladder (KUB) scans and intravenous pyelograms (IVPs). The KUB scan is carried out without contrast agent, and can detect abnormal distributions of air within the intestines, indicative of various conditions of the GI tract, and also large kidney stones. The KUB scan is usually the precursor to a follow-up imaging procedure which would entail a GI scan with barium sulphate, or an IVP if problems with the urinary system are suspected. An IVP is performed using an injected iodinated contrast agent in order to visualize the filling and emptying of the urinary system. An example of an IVP is shown in Figure 2.26. Obstruction to normal flow through the system is usually caused by kidney stones, but can result from infections of the urinary system. An IVP is carried out as a series of images acquired at different times after injection of the contrast agent. Normal excretion of the agent from the bloodstream via the kidneys takes about 30 minutes, but any obstructions can be detected or inferred from delayed passage of the contrast agent through the affected part of the urinary system.

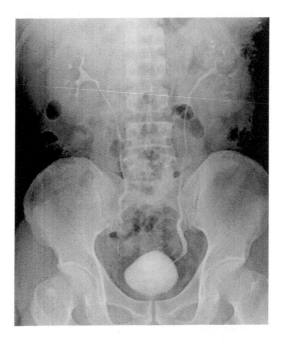

Figure 2.26

Example of an intravenous pyelogram. An iodinated contrast agent has been administered and its distribution can be seen as areas of bright signal intensity.

2.12 Computed tomography

The principles of CT were first described by Sir Godfrey Hounsfield and Allan Cormack in 1972 [4], an invention for which they were awarded jointly the Nobel Prize in Medicine in 1979. There are ~30 000 CT scanners worldwide, with more than 60 million CT scans being performed every year in the US alone. The basic principle behind CT, as shown in Figure 2.27, is that the two-dimensional structure of an object, in this case the spatially dependent X-ray attenuation coefficients, can be reconstructed from a series of one-dimensional 'projections' acquired at different angles, followed by appropriate image reconstruction, as covered in Section 1.10. A bank of solid-state detectors is situated opposite the X-ray tube and together they record a one-dimensional projection of the patient. The X-ray source and detectors are rotated through one complete revolution around the patient, with data being acquired essentially continuously. Most commercial scanners are so-called 'third generation scanners' which use a wide X-ray fan-beam and between 512 and 768 detectors. Two separate collimators are used in front of the source. The first collimator restricts the beam to an angular width of 45–60°. The second collimator, placed perpendicular to the first, restricts the beam to the desired slice thickness, typically 1–5 mm, in the patient head/foot direction. The scanner usually operates at a kVp of ~140 kV, with filtration giving an effective X-ray energy of 70–80 keV, and a tube current between 70 and 320 mA, although much higher values can be used for large patients. The focal spot size is between 0.6 and 1.6 mm. Typical operating conditions are a rotation speed of once per second, a data matrix

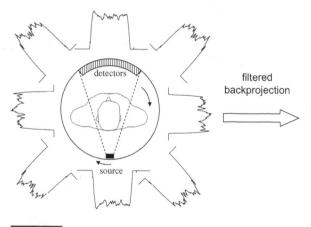
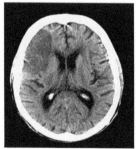

Figure 2.27

(left) The physical principle of computed tomography involves synchronous rotation of the X-ray tube and multiple detectors to record a series of one-dimensional projections. The CT image (right) is produced by the process of filtered backprojection.

of the reconstructed image of either 512×512 or 1024×1024, and a spatial resolution of ~0.35 mm.

2.12.1 Spiral / helical CT

Acquiring a single axial slice through a particular organ is of very limited diagnostic use, and so a volume consisting of multiple adjacent slices is always acquired. One way to do this is for the X-ray source to rotate once around the patient, then the patient table to be electronically moved a small distance in the head/foot direction, the X-ray source to be rotated back to its starting position, and another slice acquired. This is clearly a relatively slow process. The solution is to move the table continuously as the data are being acquired: this means that the X-ray beam path through the patient is helical, as shown in Figure 2.28. Such a scanning mode is referred to as either 'spiral' or 'helical', the two terms being interchangeable. However, there were several hardware and image processing issues that had to be solved before this concept was successfully implemented in the early 1990s. First, the very high power cables that feed the CT system cannot

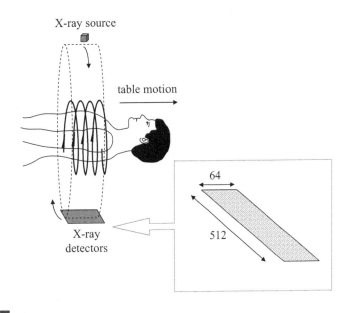

Figure 2.28

The principle of helical computed tomography in which, due to table motion along the head/foot axis, the X-ray beam plays out a helical pattern through the patient. Use of multiple detector rows (along the head/foot direction, numbers of detectors are shown for a typical 64-slice scanner) enables CT images to be acquired much more rapidly.

physically be rotated continuously in one direction, and similarly for the data transfer cables attached to the detector bank. A 'contactless' method of both delivering power and receiving data had to be designed. Second, the X-ray tube is effectively operating in continuous mode, and therefore the anode heating is much greater than for single-slice imaging. Finally, since the beam pattern through the patient is now helical rather than consisting of parallel projections, modified image reconstruction algorithms had to be developed. The first 'spiral CT', developed in the early 1990s, significantly reduced image acquisition times and enabled much greater volumes to be covered in a clinical scan.

In a helical scan, the pitch (p) is defined as the ratio of the table feed (d) per rotation of the X-ray tube to the collimated slice thickness (S):

$$p = \frac{d}{S}.$$ (2.15)

The value of p typically used in clinical scans lies between 1 and 2. The reduction in tissue radiation dose, compared to an equivalent series of single-slice scans, is equal to the value of p.

2.12.2 Multi-slice spiral CT

The efficiency of spiral CT can be increased further by incorporating an array of detectors, rather than having just a single detector, in the head/foot direction. Such an array is also shown in Figure 2.28. The increase in efficiency arises from the higher values of the table feed per rotation that can be used. Multi-slice spiral CT can be used to image larger volumes in a given time, or to image a given volume in a shorter scan time, compared to conventional spiral CT. The effective slice thickness is dictated by the dimensions of the individual detectors, rather than the collimated X-ray beam width as is the case for a single detector, which allows thinner slices to be acquired. Modern multi-detector CT (MDCT) systems have up to 256 or 320 detector rows.

2.13 Instrumentation for CT

Several components of the CT system such as the X-ray tube, collimator and anti-scatter grid are very similar to the instrumentation described previously for planar X-radiography. The tube and detectors have to be fixed to a heavy gantry, which rotates very rapidly, generating large gravitational forces. High power cables are used to deliver power to the X-ray tube, and a large parallel cable is used to transfer

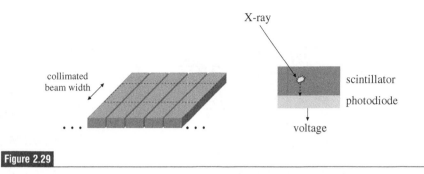

(left) A single row detector array. (right) For each solid-state detector the incident X-ray energy is converted into an electrical signal via a scintillator and photodiode.

data from the scanner to the central computer. Since each projection is acquired serially, dedicated digital signal processing boards are used to pre-process the data from each detector while the remainder of the data are being acquired, in order to speed up image reconstruction.

The detectors used in CT are solid-state devices, based upon converting the X-ray energy into light using a scintillator, and then the light being further converted into a voltage using a photodiode. The individual detector elements are typically ~15 mm in length and 1 mm wide, as shown schematically in Figure 2.29. There are several hundred of these elements in the detector module which rotates around the patient. The scintillator is based upon proprietary gadolinium ceramics, which are very effective X-ray absorbers. The anti-scatter grid is usually integrated into the detector array.

2.13.1 Instrumentation development for helical CT

A number of instrument modifications have to be made to the basic CT set-up in order to enable helical scans to be acquired. As mentioned previously, it is not possible to use fixed cables to connect either the power supply to the X-ray source, or the output of the solid state detectors directly to the digitizer and computer. Instead, multiple slip-rings are used for power and signal transmission. A slip ring is a circular contact with sliding brushes that allows the gantry to rotate continually: an example is shown in Figure 2.30.

Another equipment challenge in spiral CT scanning is that the X-rays must be produced almost continuously, without the cooling period that exists between acquisition of successive slices in conventional CT. This leads to very high temperatures at the focus of the electron beam at the surface of the anode. Anode heating is particularly problematic in abdominal scanning, which requires higher values of

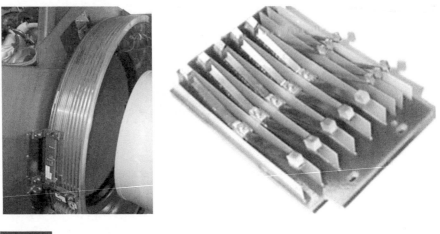

Figure 2.30

(left) A cut-away of a helical CT scanner showing the slip-rings. (right) Close-up of the sliding brushes used to transfer power from the stationary gantry to the rotating X-ray tube.

tube currents and exposures than for imaging other regions of the body. Therefore, the X-ray source must be designed to have a high heat-capacity, and very efficient cooling.

2.13.2 Detectors for multi-slice CT

In single-slice and helical CT, the slice thickness in the head/foot direction is determined by the collimated beam width in this dimension. In multi-slice CT there are up to 320 separate detectors, spanning a length of 16 cm, in the head/foot direction. Since separate signals are acquired from each of these detectors, the slice thickness is now determined by the size of the detector itself rather than the collimated beamwidth. The two-dimensional array contains the same number of circumferential elements per row as for single-detector helical CT, and so there are close to 250 000 separate signals being recorded essentially simultaneously. Examples of multi-detector modules are shown in Figure 2.31. The dimensions of the separate rows of the detectors can be the same, or they can vary in size with the smallest detectors usually being closest to the centre of the array. One such detector array, developed by Siemens, has 40 detector rows, with the 32 centre rows having 0.6 mm width, and the eight outer rows having 1.2 mm width: the total coverage is therefore 28.8 mm. In addition to being able to acquire 32 slices of 0.6 mm thickness at the centre of the array, by combining the signal from neighbouring inner elements, 24 slices of 1.2 mm thickness can also be produced. There are also

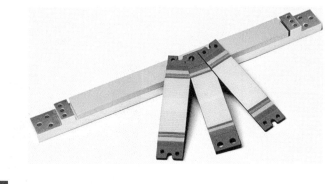

Figure 2.31

Multi-slice CT detectors, with up to 320 rows for the largest detector at the back.

methods which can improve the spatial resolution to a value smaller than the dimensions of the detector – one such is called the z-flying spot technique, in which the focal spot on the anode in the X-ray tube alternates rapidly between two slightly different positions [5].

2.14   Image reconstruction in CT

The mathematical basis for reconstruction of an image from a series of projections is the inverse Radon transform, as outlined in Section 1.10, which is performed using filtered backprojection.

2.14.1   Filtered backprojection techniques

If one assumes, for simplicity, that the signal produced in each element of the detector array arises from parallel X-rays, then the data can be filtered and backprojected to give the image. This process is illustrated in Figure 2.32 for a brain CT.

A CT image does not actually display a map of the spatially-dependent tissue attenuation coefficents per se, but rather a map of the tissue CT numbers, which are defined by:

$$CT_o = 1000 \frac{\mu_o - \mu_{H_2O}}{\mu_{H_2O}}, \qquad (2.16)$$

where CT_o is the CT number, with values expressed in Hounsfield units (HU), and μ_o the linear attenuation coefficient of the tissue in each pixel. The reconstructed

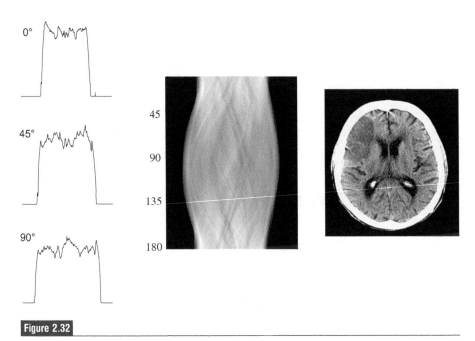

Figure 2.32

(left) Three projections acquired at different angles from a slice through the head of a patient. (centre) Sinogram showing the projections as a function of rotation angle from 0 to 180°. (right) Image produced by filtered backprojection.

Table 2.1: CT numbers of different tissues at 70 keV

Tissue	CT number (Hounsfield units)
Bone	1000–3000
Muscle	10–40
Water	0
Lipid	−50 to −100
Air	−1000
Brain (white matter)	20 to 30
Brain (grey matter)	35 to 45
Blood	40

image consists of CT numbers varying in value from +3000 to −1000. As shown in Table 2.1, the highest CT number corresponds to dense bone. Very high CT numbers also result from blood vessels containing a high dose of iodinated contrast agent, or bowel regions coated with barium sulphate. Since the attenuation coefficient of these tissues/contrast agents is very high, these regions have a high CT number and so appear bright on CT images.

2.14.2 Fan beam reconstructions

Filtered backprojection assumes that the components of the X-ray beam striking each detector element are parallel. However, as shown in Figure 2.27, the X-ray beam subtends an angle of 45–60° and, since the detector array is quite wide, the beam is far from being parallel to the detectors. The easiest way to overcome this issue, while maintaining the ability to use simple filtered backprojection, is to sort the acquired data from different projections into a set of 'synthetic projections' in which the beam geometry acts as if it were parallel to the detector. The position of the X-ray source and detectors is known with very high accuracy at each time point during the rotation, and so this process introduces negligible error into the measurements. An example of this process is shown in Figure 2.33.

2.14.3 Reconstruction of helical CT data

The helical trajectory of the X-rays through the patient means that the data do not correspond to a complete 180 or 360° rotation about the patient, and therefore the data must be resampled before filtered backprojection (incorporating fan beam resampling as explained above) can be used to produce a series of adjacent axial

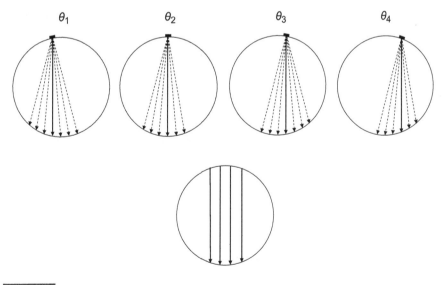

Figure 2.33

The process of data rebinning to produce parallel projections from fan beam data. Data from four different projection angles, $\theta_1 \ldots \theta_4$ are shown. One projection, shown as the solid line, is taken from each of the datasets to produce a synthetic data set (bottom) with four parallel projections, which can then use a simple filtered backprojection algorithm for image reconstruction.

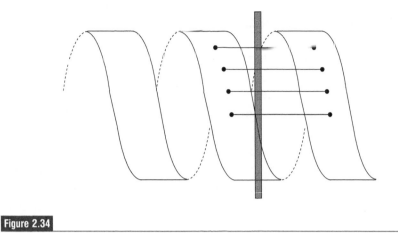

Figure 2.34

Image reconstruction from helical CT data. The process involves interpolation of data points which are not acquired. The solid dots represent acquired data, with the filled shape being the location of the interpolated data.

slices. Resampling involves linear interpolation of data points 180° apart on the spiral trajectory to estimate the 'missing' data, as shown in Figure 2.34. By adjusting the weights given to the interpolation, slices can be shifted slightly in position, and images with thicknesses greater than the collimation width can be produced by adding together adjacent reconstructed slices. These overlapping slices have been shown to increase the accuracy of lesion detection since there is less chance that a significant portion of the lesion lies between slices.

2.14.4 Reconstruction of multi-slice helical CT scans

Image reconstruction for multi-slice helical CT scans is essentially identical to that for single-slice helical scans, with the additional advantage that the slice thickness in multi-slice spiral CT can be chosen retrospectively after data acquisition. Thin slices can be reconstructed to form a high quality three-dimensional image, but the same data set can also be used to produce a set of thicker slices, with a higher SNR from each slice.

2.14.5 Pre-processing data corrections

Image reconstruction for all modes of data collection must be preceded by a series of corrections to the acquired projections to account both for instrumental imperfections and patient-induced changes in the properties of the X-ray beam. The first corrections are made for the effects of 'beam hardening', in which the effective

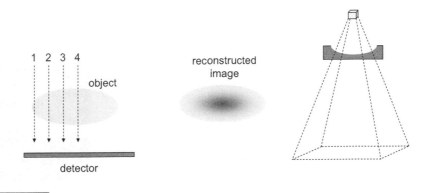

Figure 2.35

(left) Four parallel X-ray beams pass through an elliptical object with spatially uniform attenuation coefficient. The effective energy of beam 4 increases as it passes through the object to a greater degree than for beams 3, 2 and 1 since it has to travel the furthest distance through the object. This effect is known as beam hardening. An image reconstructed using filtered backprojection (centre) shows a reduced CT number in the centre of the object. (right) The effect of beam-hardening can be reduced by the use of a 'bow-tie' filter made of a metal such as aluminium, which also reduces the dose to extremities such as the arms.

energy of the X-ray beam increases as it passes through the patient, due to the greater attenuation of lower X-ray energies. This means that the effective attenuation coefficient is smaller for 'thicker' areas of the body, since the beam hardening effects are greater. In the reconstructed image, this corresponds to an apparent decrease in the CT number in the centre of the body, for example, as shown in Figure 2.35. There are a number of ways to minimize this effect, by using a 'bow-tie' filter, also shown in Figure 2.35, or by applying correction algorithms based upon the distance travelled by each X-ray beam through tissue.

The second type of correction is for slight differences in the sensitivities of individual detectors and detector channels. Imbalances in the detectors are usually measured using an object with a spatially uniform attenuation coefficent before the actual patient study. The results from this calibration scan can then be used to correct the data from the clinical scan before backprojection.

2.15 Dual-source and dual-energy CT

The temporal resolution of helical CT is basically limited by the rotation rate of the gantry. The minimum time for a 180° rotation is ~160 ms for current commercial systems. If the speed were to be increased significantly, then this would generate enormous gravitational forces on the system. An alternative method of achieving higher temporal resolutions is to add a second X-ray tube/detector into the scanner, a technique termed dual source computed tomography (DSCT). The second source

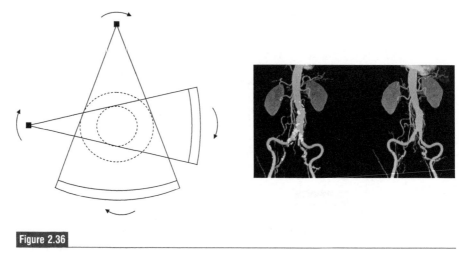

Figure 2.36

(left) A dual-source CT system. (right) Image improvement using a dual-energy CT system. The image on the left shows microcalcifications (small bright areas) superimposed on top of the arteries in a DSA scan. On the right, the microcalcifications are removed to allow accurate visualization of the arterial system.

does not cover as large a FOV as the primary source, typically about two-thirds, as shown in Figure 2.36. The temporal resolution of such a system is twice that of an equivalent single source helical CT scanner, which is particularly important for cardiac imaging [6;7].

An alternative mode of data acquisition made possible by having two different X-ray sources is to use a different kVp and tube current for each tube, thus producing 'dual-energy' images. One application is illustrated in Figure 2.36. Using a single energy, it is relatively difficult to differentiate voxels which contain bone from those with contrast agent, a clinical example being microcalcifications which are present around blood vessels which contain contrast agent. Using dual-energy imaging allows an image to be produced in which the microcalcifications are 'removed', as shown on the right of Figure 2.36. Typically, the two kVp values used are 140 keV and 80 keV, and each voxel in the image is decomposed into a percentage contribution from iodine, bone and soft-tissue.

2.16 Digital X-ray tomosynthesis

Digital X-ray tomosynthesis is a relatively new technique which might be considered as being a hybrid of planar radiography and CT [8;9]. Chest tomosynthesis is used primarily for detecting small pulmonary nodules and also for breast imaging. The patient stands in front of a flat panel detector, and a motorized unit moves the X-ray tube in a vertical path, as shown in Figure 2.37. A 0.6 mm focal spot is used,

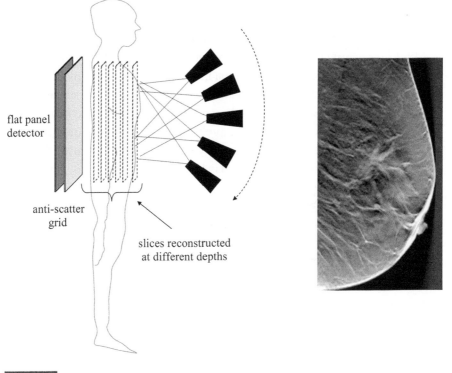

Figure 2.37

(left) The basic technique of X-ray tomosynthesis, in which an X-ray source is rotated through a relatively small angle, with planar images being formed at each angle: the digital detector remains fixed for each scan. Image reconstruction allows slices at different depths to be formed. (right) Example of a digital tomosynthesis mammogram.

with short exposure pulses of X-rays: the source-to-detector distance is ~1.8 metres. Typically 61 projection images are acquired during the vertical motion of the X-ray source. The radiation dose is much lower than for CT, but the image information content is much higher than for planar radiography. Conventional filtered backprojection algorithms cannot be used since only a limited angular coverage is acquired, so more sophisticated forms of backprojection or iterative algorithms are usually employed.

2.17 Radiation dose

The fact that X-ray imaging involves use of ionizing radiation means that there are strict safety guidelines on the single study and annual accumulated radiation doses that can be used in patients. The International Committee for Radiation Protection (ICRP) characterizes two different types of radiation effect, 'deterministic' and 'stochastic'. Deterministic effects refer to cellular damage which leads to a loss in tissue function if a sufficient number of cells are damaged. The probability of this happening is very low at low radiation doses, but climbs steadily towards unity with a dose above a certain threshold level. In contrast, stochastic effects refer to the biological situation in which the cell is not killed, but genetic mutations caused by chromosomal damage lead, in time, to development of cancer. These stochastic effects may occur at a much lower dose than deterministic effects: the higher the dose the greater the probability of cancer occurring, but importantly there is no absolute threshold level. Given that the deterministic threshold limits are far above the doses encountered in normal X-ray procedures, the greatest concern is stochastic effects.

Quantitatively, the absorbed dose (D) is defined as the radiation energy (E), measured in Joules, absorbed per kg of tissue. The value of D is given in units of grays (Gy), where 1 Gy equals 1 Joule/kg. The equivalent dose (H_T) in a tissue is given by:

$$H_T = \sum_R w_R D_{T,R}, \tag{2.17}$$

where

$$D_{T,R} = \frac{1}{m_T} \int_{m_T} D_R \, dm. \tag{2.18}$$

Note that $D_{T,R}$ is the mean absorbed dose in tissue (T) with mass (m_T) from a given amount of radiation R, and w_R is the radiation weighting factor (with a value of 1 for both X-rays and γ-rays). The unit of H_T is J/kg, but it is typically reported in sieverts (Sv), or millesieverts for realistic doses.

Some tissues are more sensitive to radiation damage than others, and this is taken into account by calculating the effective dose (E), which is given by the tissue equivalent dose weighted by the tissue weighting factor (w_T) of that organ:

$$E = \sum_T w_T H_T. \tag{2.19}$$

Values of w_T for different tissues are given in Table 2.2 with the number defined on a scale such that:

$$\sum_T w_T = 1. \tag{2.20}$$

The values of w_T represent the fraction of the total stochastic radiation risk for all the different organs and tissue. For the gonads, which have the highest risk, this

Table 2.2: Tissue weighting factors for calculations of effective dose

Tissue / organ	Tissue weighting factor, w_T
Gonads	0.2
Bone marrow (red)	0.12
Colon	0.12
Lung	0.12
Stomach	0.12
Chest	0.05
Bladder	0.05
Liver	0.05
Thyroid	0.05
Oesophagus	0.05
Average (brain, small intestines, adrenals, kidney, pancreas, muscle, spleen, thymus, uterus)	0.05
Skin	0.01
Bone surface	0.01

refers to the possibility of hereditary conditions being induced: for the other organs in Table 2.2 it refers to the risk of cancer.

In CT, the radiation dose to the patient is calculated in a slightly different way since the X-ray beam profile across each slice is not uniform, and adjacent slices receive some dose from one another. For example, in the USA the food and drug administration (FDA) defines the computed tomography dose index (CTDI) for a fourteen-slice examination to be:

$$\text{CTDI} = \frac{1}{T} \int_{-7T}^{+7T} D_z dz, \tag{2.21}$$

where D_z is the absorbed dose at position z, and T is the thickness of the slice. Since this definition has become somewhat obsolete, given the large number of slices that can be acquired on a modern CT scanner, an adapted measure is the CTDI_{100}, which is defined as:

$$\text{CTDI}_{100} = \frac{1}{NT} \int_{-5cm}^{+5cm} D_{single,z} dz, \tag{2.22}$$

where N is the number of acquired slices, and T is the nominal width of each slice. Further refinement involves the fact that the CTDI_{100} value depends upon the position within the scan plane. The weighted CTDI, CTDI_w, is defined as:

Table 2.3: Radiation doses from common planar radiography and CT scans

Procedure	Effective dose (mSv)
Abdominal planar X-ray	1.5
Chest planar X-ray	0.04
Lumbar spine planar X-ray	2.4
Intravenous pyelogram	4.6
Chest CT scan	8.3
Brain CT scan	1.8
Abdominal CT scan	7.2

$$\text{CTDI}_\text{w} = \frac{1}{3}\left(\text{CTDI}_{100}\right)_\text{centre} + \frac{2}{3}\left(\text{CTDI}_{100}\right)_\text{periphery}. \qquad (2.23)$$

For helical scans, the CTDI_vol is simply given by $\text{CTDI}_\text{w}/\text{pitch}$, where pitch was defined in Equation (2.15). All these measures are quite crude approximations, and detailed numerical simulations of CT dose for realistic patient conditions are a very active area of research, particularly with the recent advances in helical, multi-detector scanners.

Table 2.3 shows approximate doses for common X-ray procedures: the exact dose depends upon the particular system that is used for image acquisition, the patient size, etc. The limit on annual radiation dose under federal law in the USA is 50 mSv.

2.18   Clinical applications of CT

Computed tomography is used for a wide range of clinical conditions in almost every organ of the body. Brain, lymph nodes, lung, pelvis, liver, gall bladder, spleen, kidneys, GI tract, spine, and extremities are all studied using CT. The following is a very sparse survey of applications in specific areas.

2.18.1   Cerebral scans

Computed tomography is used for both chronic and acute head and brain scans. In cases of acute trauma, the radiologist looks for signs of internal bleeding, tissue oedema and skull fracture. Acute conditions can also occur, for example, if an existing aneurysm ruptures, leading to internal bleeding. Blood shows up as a high signal (high CT number) compared to the surrounding tissue, whereas oedema has a somewhat lower intensity than tissue.

Computed tomography is also used to diagnose, and follow the progression of, tumours in the brain. Meningiomas and gliomas are particularly easy to diagnose. In most cases, contrast agent is injected intravenously to highlight the tumour. In normal tissue, these agents do not cross the blood brain barrier (BBB), but tumour growth disrupts this barrier and so the agents can now enter the tumour.

2.18.2 Pulmonary disease

Normal lung tissue appears dark on CT images, but not as dark as the air within the lungs. If a focal lesion or 'nodule' is detected on a planar X-ray, then a CT is often performed. A CT scan can outline the size and geometry of the lesion much better, as well as determining whether it takes up an injected iodinated contrast agent, and whether it is calcified or not. Lung cancer, for example, typically produces nodules which have an irregular edge (caused by fibrosis surrounding the tumour), with small areas of air within the nodule. Calcification of a nodule normally indicates that it is benign rather than metastatic, with calcification producing high attenuation, and image intensities well above 100 HU. Lung cancers typically show a much greater increase in tissue attenuation than benign nodules after contrast. Lung abscesses, which are often associated with parasitic or bacterial infections, usually have a necrotic centre: this is detected by a low attenuation even after contrast agent injection, showing that there is little or no blood flow to the necrotic core. Emphysema shows up as large areas of low attenuation compared to the surrounding pulmonary parenchyma, and is usually mostly seen in the upper lobes of the lung.

2.18.3 Liver imaging

Using multi-detector CT technology, the entire liver can be imaged at high resolution within a single breath-hold. Lesions in the liver can be visualized by using dynamic imaging after iodinated contrast agent injection. A pre-contrast control scan is acquired as a baseline from which to calculate the contrast agent-induced change in image intensities. A volume of between 100 and 150 ml of contrast agent is injected over 30–40 s using a power injector. Approximately 30 s after injection, the first volume data set is acquired, which is termed the 'arterial phase' acquisition. This is used primarily to detect hypervascular lesions, which have the blood supplied by the hepatic artery: examples include focal nodular hyperplasia and hepatomas. These lesions show a greater increase in attenuation coefficient than the surrounding tissue and therefore appear brighter on the image. A second volume scan is acquired at ~65 s after injection: this is termed the 'portal phase' acquisition. This time corresponds to the enhancement of the normal liver parenchyma being at its maximum value, and therefore lesions now appear darker than the surrounding tissue. Finally, depending upon the particular study, a third data set may be acquired ~15 minutes after injection: this shows delayed enhancement of fibrotic tumours and a delayed 'fill-in' of hemangiomas.

Fatty infiltrations into liver can be caused by a number of chronic conditions including diabetes and alcoholism. The overall image intensity of liver with fatty infiltrations is typically ~20 HU lower than healthy liver, and the liver is physically enlarged. If there are specific areas of high fat infiltration, these appear as local areas of low signal intensity.

2.18.4 Cardiac imaging

Computed tomography studies of the heart normally use an iodinated contrast agent, and are primarily aimed at assessing calcifications within the heart, particularly in the coronary artery, as shown by examples in Figure 2.38. Although MRI and ultrasound scans are preferred due to the lack of ionizing radiation, in cases where pacemakers or defibrillators are present and MRI cannot be performed, then CT is useful. Calcifications of the coronary arteries are closely associated with the degree of atherosclerotic plaque formation. Even in patients without any symptoms of heart disease, the presence of coronary calcifications is highly predictive of the future development of cardiac problems. Image acquisition must be as fast as

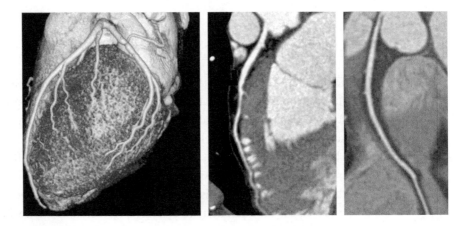

Figure 2.38

Three CT scans of the heart. (left) Three-dimensional scan from a 64-slice CT scanner shows the coronary arteries on the outside of the myocardium. (centre) and (right) Coronary angiograms of the left anterior descending artery (LAD) and right coronary artery (RCA), respectively.

possible to 'freeze' the cardiac motion and acquire all the projections within a single breath-hold if possible: image acquisition is gated to the heart motion via an ECG trigger. Although CT angiography is not a routine clinical procedure, it is very useful to rule out coronary stenoses in patients with a predisposition to the disease, and is highly informative in patients with a known or suspected congenital artery anomaly.

Exercises

The X-ray energy spectrum

2.1 Plot the energy spectra from a tungsten tube with the following kVp values: 120 keV, 80 keV, 60 keV and 40 keV.

2.2 (a) Calculate the total number of electrons bombarding the target of an X-ray tube operated at 100 mA for 0.1 seconds.

(b) Calculate the maximum energy and minimum wavelength for an X-ray beam generated at 110 kVp.

2.3 The spectrum of X-ray energies changes as the X-rays pass through tissue due to the energy dependence of the linear attenuation coefficient: this is a phenomenon known as beam hardening. A typical energy distribution of the beam from the X-ray source is shown in Figure 2.6. Sketch the energy spectrum after the beam has passed through the body.

2.4 Look up the exact binding energies of the L and M shell electrons in tungsten. Plot the exact distribution of characteristic energy lines that are produced based upon these binding energies.

2.5 Two X-ray images of the hand are shown in Figure 2.39. One corresponds to an X-ray beam with an effective energy of 140 keV and the other to an

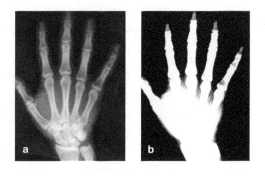

Figure 2.39

See Exercise 2.5.

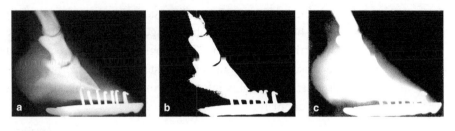

Figure 2.40

See Exercise 2.6.

effective energy of 50 keV. Explain which is which, and the reasons for the differences in image contrast and signal intensity.

2.6 Planar X-rays of a horse's leg are shown in Figure 2.40. In (a), the kVp and tube current (mA) are chosen to give high contrast between the bone and surrounding tissue. Explain how the kVp and mA settings would have to be changed (increased, decreased, remain constant) to give the images shown in (b) and (c).

2.7 Starting from Equation (2.4) derive both Equations (2.5) and (2.6).

Linear and mass attenuation coefficients

2.8 Show two mechanisms involving scattering in the body which allow Compton scattered X-rays to be detected despite the presence of an anti-scattering grid.

2.9 In Figure 2.41 calculate the X-ray intensity, as a function of the incident intensity I_0, that reaches the detector for each of the three X-ray beams. The dark-shaded area represents bone, and the light-shaded area represents tissue. The linear attenuation coefficients at the effective X-ray energy of 68 keV are $10 \ \text{cm}^{-1}$ and $1 \ \text{cm}^{-1}$ for bone and tissue, respectively.

2.10 The linear attenuation coefficient of a gadolinium-based phosphor used for detection of X-rays is $560 \ \text{cm}^{-1}$ at an X-ray energy of 150 keV. What percentage of X-rays are detected by phosphor layers of 10 μm, 25 μm, and 50 μm thickness? What are the trade-offs in terms of spatial resolution?

X-ray detectors

2.11 An X-ray with energy 60 keV strikes a gadolinium-based phosphor on a CR plate producing photons at a wavelength of 415 nm. The energy conversion coefficient for this process is 20%. How many photons are produced for each incident X-ray? (Planck's constant $= 6.63 \times 10^{34}$ Js, 1 eV$=1.602 \times 10^{-19}$J).

2.12 An X-ray is Compton scattered by an angle θ at a distance z from the top of the anti-scatter grid. Using simple geometry, calculate the maximum value of θ for a given grid ratio h/d that results in the X-ray being detected.

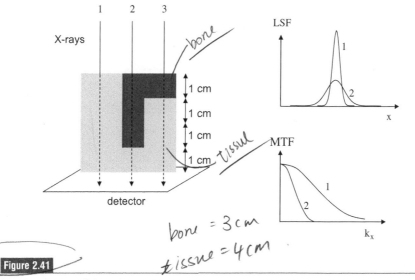

Figure 2.41

See Exercises 2.9 (left) and 2.15 (right).

Quantitative characteristics of planar X-ray images

2.13 The width of the electron beam in an X-ray tube is 6 mm, and the anode bevel angle is 10°. The patient is placed 180 cm from the X-ray tube, directly on top of the flat panel detector. Calculate the geometric unsharpness for a very small lesion at the front of the abdomen and at the back of the abdomen, assuming that the tissue thickness of the body at this point is 25 cm.

2.14 If the average number of X-rays striking the detector is 100 per pixel per second, what is the probability that only 90 strike in any one second? If the X-ray dose is increased by a factor of ten, what is the probability of 900 striking?

2.15 (a) Match up a thick and thin phosphor layer in computed radiography with its associated LSF (1 or 2) in Figure 2.41.

(b) Similarly, match up a small and large X-ray focal spot with its MTF (1 or 2). Provide a brief explanation for each choice.

Specialized X-ray imaging methods

2.16 In mammographic examinations, the breast is compressed between two plates. Answer the following with a brief explanation.

(a) Is the geometric unsharpness increased or decreased by compression?

(b) Why is the image contrast improved by this procedure?

(c) Is the required X-ray dose for a given image SNR higher or lower with compression?

2.17 In digital subtraction angiography, two images are acquired, the first before injection of the contrast agent, and the other post-injection.

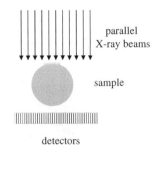

Figure 2.42

See Exercise 2.18.

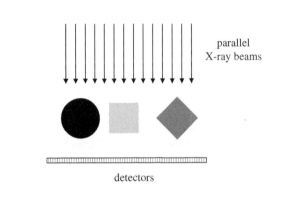

Figure 2.43

See Exercise 2.20.

(a) Write an expression for the X-ray intensity (I_1) in the first scan in terms of I_0, μ_{tissue}, x_{tissue}, μ_{blood} and x_{vessel}, where x_{tissue} and x_{vessel} are the dimensions of the respective organs in the direction of X-ray propagation.

(b) Write a corresponding expression for the X-ray intensity (I_2) for the second scan, replacing μ_{blood} with $\mu_{constrast}$

(c) Is the image signal intensity from static tissue removed by subtracting the two images?

(d) Show that the signal from static tissue is removed by computing the quantity $\log(I_2)-\log(I_1)$.

Computed tomography

2.18 Draw the CT projection obtained from the set-up shown in Figure 2.42. Assume that the spherical sample has a uniform attenuation coefficient throughout its volume.

2.19 Considering the effects of beam hardening, draw the actual CT projection that would be obtained from the object shown in Figure 2.42. Sketch the final

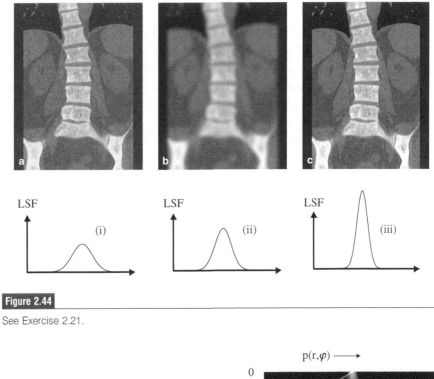

Figure 2.44

See Exercise 2.21.

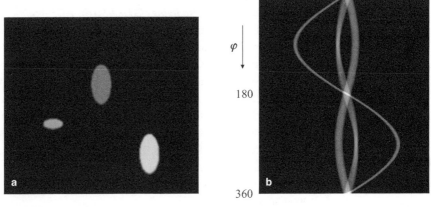

Figure 2.45

See Exercises 2.22 (a) and 2.23 (b).

image that would be formed from filtered backprojection of all of the projections acquired in a full scan of the sample in Exercise 2.18.

2.20 For the object shown in Figure 2.43, draw the projections that would be acquired at angles $\varphi=0$, 45, 90, 135 and 180° (ignore beam hardening). Sketch the sinogram for values of φ from 0 to 360°.

2.21 Shown in Figure 2.44 are three CT images: one represents the reconstructed image with no filtering, one has been high-pass filtered and the other has been low-pass filtered. For each image, (a), (b) and (c), state which form of filtering has been used, and the effects on signal-to-noise, spatial resolution, and contrast-to-noise of the filtering. Finally, match the image to one of the line spread functions, (i), (ii), or (iii).

2.22 For the CT image shown in Figure 2.45(a), sketch the sinogram that produced such an image.

2.23 For the sinogram in Figure 2.45(b), sketch the filtered backprojection image that would result.

References

[1] Cowen AR, Davies AG and Kengyelics SM. Advances in computed radiography systems and their physical imaging characteristics. *Clinical Radiology* 2007;**62**(12), 1132–41.

[2] Cowen AR, Kengyelics SM and Davies AG. Solid-state, flat-panel, digital radiography detectors and their physical imaging characteristics. *Clinical Radiology* 2008;**63**(5), 487–98.

[3] Cowen AR, Davies AG and Sivananthan MU. The design and imaging characteristics of dynamic, solid-state, flat-panel X-ray image detectors for digital fluoroscopy and fluorography. *Clinical Radiology* 2008;**63**(10), 1073–85.

[4] Hounsfield GN. Computerized transverse axial scanning (Tomography).1. Description of system. *British Journal of Radiology* 1973;**46**(552), 1016–22.

[5] Flohr T, Stierstorfer K, Ulzheimer S *et al.* Image reconstruction and image quality evaluation for a 64-slice CT scanner with z-flying focal spot. *Medical Physics* 2005:**32**, 2536–47.

[6] Flohr TG, Bruder H, Stierstorfer K *et al.* Image reconstruction and image quality evaluation for a dual source CT scanner. *Medical Physics* 2008;**35**(12), 5882–97.

[7] Petersilka M, Bruder H, Krauss B, Stierstorfer K and Flohr TG. Technical principles of dual source CT. *Eur J Radiol* 2008 Dec;**68**(3), 362–8.

[8] Dobbins JT. Tomosynthesis imaging: At a translational crossroads. *Medical Physics* 2009;**36**(6), 1956–67.

[9] Dobbins JT, III and McAdams HP. Chest tomosynthesis: Technical principles and clinical update. *Eur J Radiol* 2009 Jul 17.

3 Nuclear medicine: Planar scintigraphy, SPECT and PET/CT

3.1 Introduction

In nuclear medicine scans a very small amount, typically nanogrammes, of radioactive material called a radiotracer is injected intravenously into the patient. The agent then accumulates in specific organs in the body. How much, how rapidly and where this uptake occurs are factors which can determine whether tissue is healthy or diseased and the presence of, for example, tumours. There are three different modalities under the general umbrella of nuclear medicine. The most basic, planar scintigraphy, images the distribution of radioactive material in a single two-dimensional image, analogous to a planar X-ray scan. These types of scan are mostly used for whole-body screening for tumours, particularly bone and metastatic tumours. The most common radiotracers are chemical complexes of technetium (^{99m}Tc), an element which emits mono-energetic γ-rays at 140 keV. Various chemical complexes of ^{99m}Tc have been designed in order to target different organs in the body. The second type of scan, single photon emission computed tomography (SPECT), produces a series of contiguous two-dimensional images of the distribution of the radiotracer using the same agents as planar scintigraphy. There is, therefore, a direct analogy between planar X-ray/CT and planar scintigraphy/SPECT. A SPECT scan is most commonly used for myocardial perfusion, the so-called 'nuclear cardiac stress test'. The final method is positron emission tomography (PET). This involves injection of a different type of radiotracer, one which emits positrons (positively charged electrons). These annihilate with electrons within the body, emitting γ-rays with an energy of 511 keV. The PET method has by far the highest sensitivity of the three techniques, producing high quality three-dimensional images with particular emphasis on oncological diagnoses. Within the past five years PET and CT systems have been integrated such that all commercial units sold are now combined PET/CT scanners. A PET/CT system requires a small cyclotron to be situated on-site and therefore only relatively large hospitals have one, whereas SPECT systems are very widely available and planar scintigraphy is ubiquitous. There are between 15 and 20 million nuclear medicine scans performed annually in the USA, with SPECT comprising approximately

75% of the total (of these ~60% are for myocardial perfusion). The number of PET/CT scans is ~2 million, but has roughly doubled every year for the past five years.

Figure 3.1 shows the basic form of the gamma camera which is used in both planar scintigraphy and SPECT. In planar scintigraphy a single gamma camera is held stationary above the patient. In SPECT either two or three cameras are rotated slowly around the patient with data collected at each angular increment. Decay of the radiotracer within the body produces γ-rays, a small percentage of which pass through the body (the vast majority are absorbed in the body). A two-dimensional collimator (similar to the anti-scatter grid in X-ray imaging) is placed between the patient and the detector, so that only those γ-rays which strike the gamma camera at a perpendicular angle are detected. A large, single scintillation crystal is used to convert the energy of the γ-rays into light, which is in turn converted into an electrical signal by high-gain photomultiplier tubes (PMTs). Spatial information is encoded in the current produced by each PMT via a resistor-based positioning network, or its digital equivalent in more modern systems. A pulse-height analyzer is used to reject signals from γ-rays that have been Compton scattered in the body and therefore contain no useful signal. Finally, the signal is digitized and displayed.

Relative to most other imaging modalities, nuclear medicine scans (in particular planar scintigraphy and SPECT) are characterized as having a poor SNR, low spatial resolution (~5–10 mm) and slow image acquisition, but extremely high sensitivity (being able to detect nanograms of injected radioactive material), and very high specificity since there is no natural radioactivity from the body. Due to

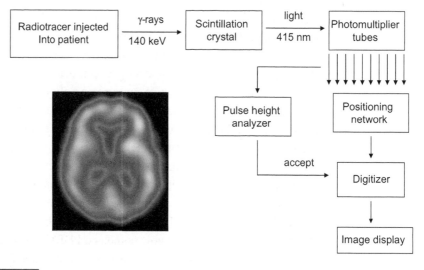

Figure 3.1

The operation of a nuclear medicine gamma camera. The inset shows a SPECT brain scan using ^{99m}Tc.

the intrinsic functional characteristics of the information content of the images, nuclear medicine is an important complement to MRI, CT and ultrasound.

3.2 Radioactivity and radiotracer half-life

A radioactive isotope is one which undergoes a spontaneous change in the composition of the nucleus, termed a 'disintegration', resulting in emission of energy. Radioactivity is given the symbol Q, and is defined as the number of disintegrations per second, or alternatively the time rate of change of the number of radioactive nuclei. For N nuclei of a particular radioactive isotope, then:

$$Q = -\frac{dN}{dt} = \lambda N, \tag{3.1}$$

where λ is defined as the decay constant and has units of s^{-1}. Radioactivity is measured in units of curies (Ci), where one curie equals 3.7×10^{10} disintegrations per second. Historically, this is the number of disintegrations per second from 1 gramme of radium and is named after Pierre Curie. For doses relevant to clinical nuclear medicine studies, the most common units are millicuries (mCi), 1/1000 of a curie or 3.7×10^7 disintegrations per second. Equation (3.1) can be solved to give:

$$N(t) = N(t = 0)e^{-\lambda t}. \tag{3.2}$$

One of the most common measures of radioactivity is the half-life ($\tau_{1/2}$), which is the time required for the radioactivity to drop to one-half of its value, as shown in Figure 3.2. From Figure 3.2 it is clear that the value of $\tau_{1/2}$ is independent of the

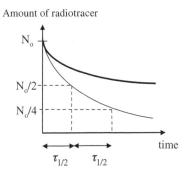

Figure 3.2

A plot of the amount of two different radiotracers as a function of time. The thin line corresponds to a radiotracer with a shorter half-life than the one indicated by the thick line. The $\tau_{1/2}$ refers to the radiotracer with the shorter half-life.

value of N. Since the value of λ is also independent of N, $\tau_{1/2}$ also corresponds to the time for the number of radioactive nuclei to drop by half, and so from Equation (3.2) the value of $\tau_{1/2}$ is given by.

$$\tau_{1/2} = \frac{\ln 2}{\lambda}. \tag{3.3}$$

In nuclear medicine scans the total radioactive dose experienced by the patient is limited by federal safely guidelines. To calculate the dose, the biological half-life of the radiotracer (how long the radiotracer remains in the body) must also be considered. In many cases, excretion of the radiotracer from tissue is an exponential decay which can be characterized by a corresponding biological half-life, $\tau_{1/2,\text{bio}}$. The effective half-life ($\tau_{1/2,\text{eff}}$) of the radioactivity within the body is a combination of the two half-lives and is given by:

$$\tau_{1/2,\text{eff}} = \frac{\tau_{1/2}\tau_{1/2,\text{bio}}}{\tau_{1/2} + \tau_{1/2,\text{bio}}}. \tag{3.4}$$

Therefore, the value of $\tau_{1/2,\text{eff}}$ is always less than the shorter of the two half-lives, $\tau_{1/2}$ and $\tau_{1/2,\text{bio}}$.

Example 3.1   Two patients undergo nuclear medicine scans. One receives a dose of radiotracer A and the other radioatracer B. The half-life of A is 6 hours and of B is 24 hours. If the administered dose of radiotracer A is three times that of radiotracer B, and the biological half-lives of A and B are 6 and 12 hours respectively, at what time is the radioactivity in the body the same for the two patients?

Solution   Mathematically we can solve the following for the time t:

$$3e^{-t\lambda_A} = e^{-t\lambda_B}.$$

The values of λ_A and λ_B can be derived from Equation (3.4) and are 6.42×10^{-5} and 2.41×10^{-5} s^{-1}, respectively. Solving for t gives a value of 7.63 hours.

3.3 Properties of radiotracers for nuclear medicine

The ideal properties of a radiotracer for planar scintigraphy and SPECT include:

(i) A radioactive half-life that is short enough to produce significant radioactivity without requiring a very large initial dose, but not so short that there is significant decay before the required post-injection delay to allow the radiotracer to clear the blood and distribute in the relevant organs.

(ii) Decay should be via emission of a mono-energetic γ-ray without emission of alpha- or beta-particles. A mono-energetic γ-ray allows discrimination between Compton scattered and unscattered γ-rays, thereby improving image contrast. Alpha- or beta-particles are completely absorbed within tissue, therefore increasing the radioactive dose without giving any useful image information.

(iii) The energy of the γ-ray should be greater than ~100 keV so that a reasonable proportion of γ-rays which are emitted deep within the tissue have sufficient energy to travel through the body and reach the detector.

(iv) The energy of the γ-ray should be less than ~200 keV so that the rays do not penetrate the thin lead septa in the collimator (which is analogous to the anti-scatter grid in X-ray imaging).

(v) The radiotracer should have a high uptake in the organ of interest and relatively low non-specific uptake in the rest of the body. These two factors lower the required dose for the patient and increase the image contrast, respectively.

The most widely used radiotracer is ^{99m}Tc which is involved in over 90% of planar scintigraphy and SPECT studies. It exists in a metastable state, i.e. one with a reasonably long half-life (6.02 hours), and is formed from ^{99}Mo according to the decay scheme

$$^{99}_{42}\text{Mo} \xrightarrow{\tau_{1/2}\,=\,66\,\text{hours}} {}^{0}_{1}\beta + {}^{99m}_{43}\text{Tc} \xrightarrow{\tau_{1/2}\,=\,6\,\text{hours}} {}^{99g}_{43}\text{Tc} + \gamma.$$

The energy of the emitted γ-ray is 140 keV. It is important to note that this is a mono-energetic emission, unlike the wide spectrum of energies of X-rays produced by an X-ray source covered in Chapter 2. The on-site generation and use of ^{99m}Tc are discussed in detail in Section 3.4.

Note that γ-rays can also be produced via a process termed electron capture, in which an orbital electron from the K or L shell is 'captured' by the nucleus. Electrons from the outer shells fill the gap in the K or L shell in a cascade process. The difference in energy between the respective energy levels is released as γ-rays of a characteristic energy. Several useful radiotracers decay via this mechanism: examples include iodine-123, thallium-201 and indium-111. Table 3.1 lists properties of the most commonly used radiotracers in nuclear medicine.

3.4   The technetium generator

A technetium generator is delivered to a nuclear medicine department at the beginning of the week, and is returned at the end of the week. It is a very convenient method for producing ^{99m}Tc. An on-site technetium generator comprises an

Table 3.1: Properties of common radiotracers used in planar scintigraphy and SPECT

Radiotracer	Half-life (hours)	γ-ray energy (keV)	Clinical application
^{99m}Tc	6.0	140	various
^{67}Ga	76.8	93, 185, 300, 394	tumour detection
^{201}Tl	72	167, 68–82 (X-rays)	myocardial viability
^{133}Xe	127.2	81	lung ventilation
^{111}In	67.2	171, 245	inflammation

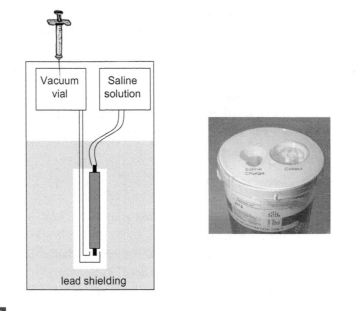

Figure 3.3

(left) A technetium generator. (right) A commercial technetium generator.

alumina ceramic column with radioactive ^{99}Mo absorbed on to its surface in the form of ammonium molybdate, $(NH_4)_2MoO_4$. The column is housed within a lead shield for safety. A schematic and photograph of a Tc-generator are shown in Figure 3.3. As outlined previously, the ^{99}Mo decays into ^{99m}Tc which in turn decays into ^{99g}Tc, the ground state of Tc . At any given time the generator column contains a mixture of ^{99}Mo, ^{99m}Tc and ^{99g}Tc. To remove the ^{99m}Tc selectively a vial with physiological saline is placed at the input to the column and a needle and empty vial at the outlet. The saline is drawn through the column and washes out most of the ^{99m}Tc which does not bind strongly to the column and is eluted in the form of sodium pertechnetate: roughly 80% of the available ^{99m}Tc is eluted compared to less than 1% of the ^{99}Mo. Appropriate radioassays are then carried out to determine the concentration and purity of the eluted ^{99m}Tc, with Al and ^{99}Mo impurities required to be below certain safety levels. Typically, the technetium is eluted every 24 hours, and the generator is replaced once a week. Most nuclear medicine scans are therefore scheduled for the beginning of a week.

The time-dependence of the radioactivity can be analyzed as a two-step process. The number of ^{99}Mo atoms, denoted by N_1, decreases with time from an initial maximum value N_0 at time $t = 0$. This radioactive decay produces N_2 atoms of ^{99m}Tc, which decay to form N_3 atoms of ^{99g}Tc, the final stable product:

$$^{99}\text{Mo} \xrightarrow{\lambda_1} \, ^{99m}\text{Tc} \xrightarrow{\lambda_2} \, ^{99g}\text{Tc}$$
$$(N_1) \qquad (N_2) \qquad (N_3)$$

The values of λ_1 and λ_2, derived from the respective half-lives, are 2.92×10^{-6} s^{-1} and 3.21×10^{-5} s^{-1}, respectively. The decay of the ^{99}Mo (termed the parent nucleus) is given by Equation (3.2), $N_1 = N_0 e^{-\lambda_1 t}$. Since there is a two-step decay process, the amount of ^{99m}Tc increases due to the decay of ^{99}Mo, but decreases due to its own decay to ^{99g}Tc:

$$\frac{dN_2}{dt} = \lambda_1 N_1 - \lambda_2 N_2 \Rightarrow \frac{dN_2}{dt} + \lambda_2 N_2 = \lambda_1 N_1. \tag{3.5}$$

There are a number of methods for solving this simple first order differential equation. For example, the homogeneous and particular equations can be solved:

$$\begin{aligned} \text{(homogeneous)}\; N_2 &= C e^{-\lambda_2 t} \\ \text{(particular)}\; N_2 &= D e^{-\lambda_1 t} \end{aligned} \tag{3.6}$$

For the particular solution, solving for D gives:

$$D = \frac{\lambda_1 N_0}{\lambda_2 - \lambda_1}. \tag{3.7}$$

Adding together the homogeneous and particular solutions:

$$N_2 = C e^{-\lambda_2 t} + \frac{\lambda_1 N_0}{\lambda_2 - \lambda_1} e^{-\lambda_1 t}. \tag{3.8}$$

Since we know that $N_2 = 0$ at $t = 0$, using this boundary condition we can solve for the constant C:

$$C = -\frac{\lambda_1 N_0}{\lambda_2 - \lambda_1}. \tag{3.9}$$

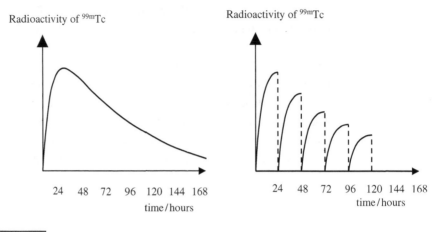

Figure 3.4

(left) Theoretical plot of the radioactivity of ^{99m}Tc vs time for a generator that is not milked. (right) Practical radioactivity curve in which the generator is milked every 24 hours, as shown by the dashed lines.

The final solution for N_2 is therefore:

$$N_2 = \frac{\lambda_1 N_0}{\lambda_2 - \lambda_1} \left(e^{-\lambda_1 t} - e^{-\lambda_2 t} \right). \tag{3.10}$$

The radioactivity, Q_2, of ^{99m}Tc is therefore given by:

$$Q_2 = \lambda_2 N_2 = \frac{\lambda_1 \lambda_2 N_0}{\lambda_2 - \lambda_1} \left(e^{-\lambda_1 t} - e^{-\lambda_2 t} \right). \tag{3.11}$$

As might have been intuitively expected, the radioactivity is proportional to the difference of two exponentials, one governing the increase in the amount of ^{99m}Tc and the other its decay. Figure 3.4 shows that the maximum value of the radioactivity occurs at ~24 hours, which is therefore the logical time at which the generator is first 'milked', i.e. the ^{99m}Tc is removed. The radioactivity drops to zero and then begins to increase again. Maximum levels of radioactivity occur roughly every 24 hours, which makes it very easy to incorporate into a daily clinical schedule.

3.5 The distribution of technetium-based radiotracers within the body

The ^{99m}Tc eluted from the generator is in the form of sodium pertechnetate, NaTcO$_4$. This compound is not widely used for nuclear medicine scans, with its most common application being to GI tract bleeding in young children. Further chemical modification is needed to produce the most commonly used radiotracers. In general, a strong chemical bond must be formed between a chemical ligand and the Tc ion such that the body is protected from the 'raw' metal ion. The ligand must bind the metal ion tightly so that the radiotracer does not fragment in the body. The particular ligand is also chosen to have high selectivity for the organ of interest. General factors which effect the biodistribution of a particular agent include the strength of the binding to blood proteins such as human serum albumin (HSA), the lipophilicity and ionization of the chemical ligand (since transport across membranes is fastest for lipophilic and non-ionized species), and the means of excretion from the body e.g. via the liver or kidneys.

Chemical modification is performed using special kits which are provided by different manufacturers. Two of the most common radiotracers are Ceretec, used for measuring cerebral perfusion, and Sestamibi, used for evaluation of myocardial perfusion. The Ceretec kit contains a pre-dispensed freeze-dried mixture of the ligand exametazime, stannous chloride dihydrate as a reducing agent and 4.5 mg sodium chloride, sealed under nitrogen atmosphere. When the sodium pertechnetate/saline solution from the ^{99}Tc generator is added to the vial of Ceretec, a ^{99m}Tc complex with exametazime is formed which is injected i.v. into the patient within 30 minutes.

3.6   The gamma camera

The gamma camera, shown in Figure 3.5, is the instrumental basis for both planar scintigraphy and SPECT [1]. The patient lies on a bed beneath the gamma camera, which is positioned close to the organ of interest. The gamma camera must be capable of γ-ray detection rates of up to tens of thousands per second, should reject those γ-rays that have been scattered in the body and therefore have no useful spatial information, and must have as high a sensitivity as possible in order to produce the highest quality images within a clinically acceptable imaging time. The roles of each of the separate components of the gamma camera are covered in the following sections.

3.6.1   The collimator

The role of the collimator in nuclear medicine is very similar to that of the anti-scatter grid in X-ray imaging. Since γ-rays from a source of radioactivity within the body are emitted in all directions, a much higher degree of collimation is required

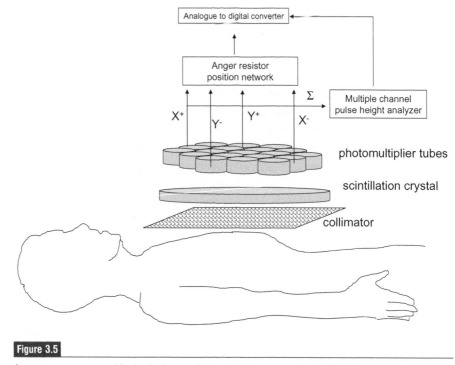

Figure 3.5

A gamma camera used for both planar scintigraphy (one camera) and SPECT (two or three rotating cameras).

in nuclear medicine than in X-ray imaging. This, together with the high attenuation of γ-rays within the body, leads to a very high proportion of emitted γ-rays ($>99.9\%$) not being detected. There are six basic collimator designs: parallel hole, slanthole, converging, diverging, fan-beam and pinhole. Each has particular properties in terms of effects on image SNR, CNR and spatial resolution. The parallel hole collimator is the most common design, and so is described first.

(i) *Parallel hole collimator.* As the name suggests, all the holes in the collimator are parallel to each other. The collimator is usually constructed from thin strips of lead in a hexagonally-based 'honeycomb' geometry, although round holes in a hexagonal array can also be used. Ideally there would be zero transmission of γ-rays through the septa themselves, but since this is not possible the septa are designed so that 95% of γ-rays are attenuated. Due to the finite transmission of γ-rays through the septa, the effective septal length (L_{eff}) is slightly shorter than the actual physical length (L) of the septa, and is given by:

$$L_{eff} = L - \frac{2}{\mu_{septa}}.$$ (3.12)

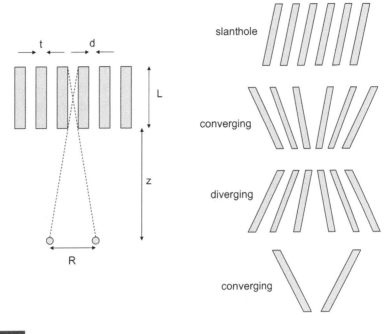

(left) A parallel hole collimator, with parameters necessary to calculate the spatial resolution, R. The patient would be positioned at the bottom of the figure, with the gamma camera at the top. (right) Four common types of collimator: from top-to-bottom, slanting hole, converging, diverging and pinhole.

The dimensions and separation of the lead strips also determine the contribution made by the collimator to the overall spatial resolution of the gamma camera. In Figure 3.6, if two point sources are located a distance less than R apart they cannot be resolved. The value of R, the spatial resolution, is given by:

$$R = \frac{d(L_{eff} + z)}{L_{eff}}. \tag{3.13}$$

An important fact to note from Equation (3.13) is that the spatial resolution of the image depends upon the depth (z) within the body of the organ in which the radiotracer source accumulates. Regions of radioactivity closer to the surface produce a better spatial resolution than those deeper in the body, and this fact must be taken into account for image interpretation.

Equation (3.13) also shows that the spatial resolution can be improved by increasing the length of the septa in the collimator, decreasing the septal thickness, and/or positioning the gamma camera as close to the patient as possible. However, the values of L and d also affect the collimator efficiency, which is defined as the fraction of γ-rays detected divided by the total number emitted (ignoring attenuation in the body). The efficiency (g) of the detector is given by:

$$g \approx K^2 \frac{d^2}{L_{eff}^2} \frac{d^2}{(d+t)^2}, \qquad (3.14)$$

where the value of K depends upon the particular hole-geometry and has a value of 0.26 for hexagonal holes in a hexagonal array. It is clear from Equation (3.14) that there is an intrinsic trade-off between spatial resolution and collimator efficiency.

Collimators used for ^{99m}Tc imaging are referred to as low-energy (140 keV γ-rays): those with relatively large holes are termed low-energy all-purpose (LEAP) and those with smaller holes and longer septa are called low-energy high-resolution (LEHR). Medium energy and high energy collimators have septa of increasing thickness and are used for ^{67}Ga/^{111}In and ^{131}I, respectively.

(ii) *Slanthole collimators* consist of parallel septa which are all tilted at the same angle with respect to the detection crystal. They are used primarily for breast and cardiac imaging.

(iii) *Converging collimators* have the holes focused towards the body, with the centre of curvature ideally located at the middle of the imaging field-of-view (FOV). A converging collimator is used to magnify the image and increase the spatial resolution.

(iv) *A diverging collimator* is essentially a converging collimator that has been turned around. This enables a larger FOV, compared to a parallel hole collimator, to be imaged. One application is planar scintigraphy of the whole body.

(v) *Fan-beam collimators* are used primarily for brain and heart studies. The two dimensions of the collimator have different geometries: in the head/foot direction the holes are parallel, whereas in the radial direction they are similar to a converging collimator. Thus, these types of collimator provide image magnification over a reduced FOV.

(vi) *Pinhole collimators* are used for imaging very small organs such as the thyroid and parathyroid. These collimators have a single hole with interchangeable inserts that come with a 3, 4 or 6 mm aperture. A pinhole collimator produces an image with significant magnification and higher spatial resolution, but also produces geometric distortion, particularly at the edges of the image.

3.6.2   The detector scintillation crystal and coupled photomultiplier tubes

γ-rays not attenuated in the body are detected using a scintillation crystal which converts their energy into light. In the gamma camera, the detector is a large single crystal of thallium-activated sodium iodide, NaI(Tl), approximately 40–50 cm diameter. When a γ-ray strikes the crystal, it loses energy through photoelectric and Compton interactions which result in a population of excited electronic states within the crystal. De-excitation of these states occurs ~230 nanoseconds later via emission of photons with a wavelength of 415 nm (visible blue light), corresponding to a photon energy of ~4 eV. A very important characteristic of scintillators such as NaI(Tl) is that the amount of light (the number of photons) produced is directly proportional to the energy of the incident γ-ray.

Sodium iodide is chosen for a number of reasons: (i) it has a high linear attenuation coefficient of 2.22 cm^{-1} at 140 keV , (ii) it is efficient with one light photon produced per 30 eV of energy absorbed, an efficiency of ~15%, (iii) it is transparent to its own light emission at 415 nm and so little energy is lost due to absorption, (iv) large circular or rectangular crystals can be grown easily and inexpensively, and (v) the 415 nm emission wavelength is well-matched to the optimal performance of conventional photomultiplier tubes (PMTs). The only disadvantage of a NaI(Tl) crystal is that it is hygroscopic (absorbs water) and so must be hermetically sealed, therefore also making it quite mechanically fragile.

The thickness of the crystal involves the same trade-off between spatial resolution and sensitivity as for a DR detector in planar X-ray imaging: the thicker the crystal the broader is the light spread function and the lower the spatial resolution, but the greater the number of γ-rays detected and the higher the SNR. For imaging with ^{99m}Tc or ^{201}Tl, the optimal crystal thickness is ~6 mm. However, although the vast majority of nuclear medicine scans use ^{99m}Tc, the gamma camera is also used for other radiotracers such as ^{68}Ga, ^{131}I and ^{111}In which emit higher γ-ray energies and require a thicker crystal, and so a compromise crystal thickness of 1 cm is generally used. Figure 3.7 shows rectangular NaI(Tl) crystals produced commercially for gamma cameras, as well as the steep drop-off in the value of μ as a function of γ-ray energy for such crystals.

For every γ-ray that hits the scintillation crystal a few thousand photons are produced, each with a very low energy of a few electronvolts. These very low light signals need to be amplified and converted into an electrical current that can be digitized: PMTs are the devices used for this specific task. The basic design of a PMT is shown in Figure 3.8. The inside surface of the transparent entrance window of the PMT is coated with a material such as caesium antimony (CsSb) which forms a photocathode. Free electrons (photoelectrons) are generated via photoelectric interactions when the photons from the scintillation crystal strike this material. These electrons are accelerated towards the first stage of amplification, a metal plate termed a dynode held at a voltage of +300 volts with respect to the photocathode. This plate is also coated with a bialkali material such as CsSb. When the electrons strike this dynode several secondary electrons are emitted for every incident electron: a typical amplification factor is between 3 and 6. A series of

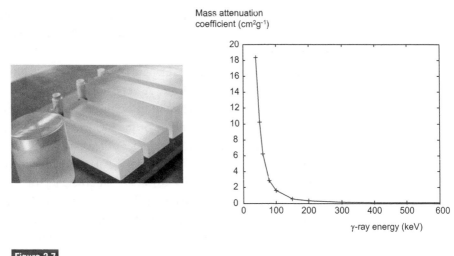

Mass attenuation coefficient (cm^2g^{-1})

γ-ray energy (keV)

Figure 3.7

(left) Commercially produced crystals of NaI(Tl). (right) Plot of the mass attenuation coefficient for NaI(Tl) vs. γ-ray energy, showing an approximately exponential decrease with increasing energy.

eight to ten further accelerating dynodes, each at a voltage of +100 volts with respect to the previous one, produces between 10^5 and 10^6 electrons for each initial photoelectron, creating an amplified current at the output of the PMT. A high voltage power supply is required for each PMT, in the range 1–2 kV. The PMTs are sealed in glass, and the entire enclosure evacuated to reduce attenuation of the electrons between the dynodes: a photograph of a single PMT is shown in Figure 3.8.

Since each PMT has a diameter of 2–3 cm, and the NaI(Tl) crystal is much larger in size, a number of PMTs are closely coupled to the scintillation crystal. The most efficient packing geometry is hexagonally-close-packed, which also has the property that the distance from the centre of one PMT to that of each neighbouring PMT is the same: this property is important for determination of the spatial location of the scintillation event using an Anger position network, as covered in the following section. Arrays of 61, 75 or 91 PMTs are typically used, with a thin optical coupling layer used to interface the surface of each PMT with the scintillation crystal. Each PMT should ideally have an identical energy response, i.e. the output current for a given γ-ray energy should be the same. If this is not the case, then artifacts are produced in the image. For planar nuclear medicine scans, a variation in uniformity of up to 10% can be tolerated; however, for SPECT imaging, covered later in this chapter, this value should be less than 1%. In practice, calibration of the PMTs is performed using samples of uniform and known radioactivity, and automatic data correction algorithms can then be applied to the data. More recently, continuous monitoring of individual PMTs during a nuclear

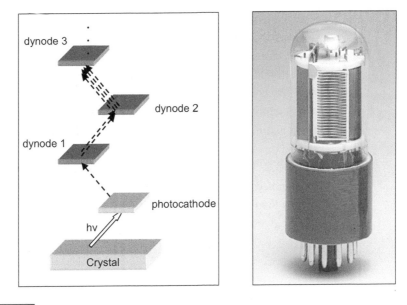

Figure 3.8

(left). The first three amplification stages in a PMT tube. (right) A commercial PMT.

medicine scan has become possible using a light-emitting diode (LED) calibration source for each PMT.

Example 3.2   The linear attenuation coefficients for a NaI(Tl) crystal for the radiotracer elements ^{99m}Tc, ^{68}Ga, ^{131}I and ^{111}In are 2.2, 1.7, 1.3 and 1.2 cm^{-1}, respectively. For 6 mm and 1 cm thickness crystals, calculate the relative signal intensities for each radiotracer element.

Solution   The relative values can be calculated as $(1-e^{-\mu x})$, noting that the signal intensities are proportional to the number of γ-rays *absorbed* and not passing through the crystal. If we take values relative to 1, corresponding to all of the γ-rays being *absorbed,* this gives values of: (6 mm crystal) 0.73, 0.64, 0.54 and 0.51, (1 cm crystal) 0.89, 0.82, 0.73 and 0.7. Note the greater proportional increase in sensitivity for the higher energy radionuclides for the 1 cm thickness crystal compared to the 6 mm.

3.6.3 The Anger position network and pulse height analyzer

Whenever a scintillation event occurs in a NaI(Tl) crystal the PMT closest to the scintillation event produces the largest output current. If this were the only method of signal localization, then the spatial resolution would be no finer than the dimensions of the PMT, i.e., several cm. However, adjacent PMTs produce smaller output currents, with the amount of light detected being approximately inversely proportional to the distance between the scintillation events and the particular PMT. By comparing the magnitudes of the currents from all the PMTs, the location of the scintillation within the crystal can be much better estimated. In older analogue gamma cameras this process was carried out using an Anger logic circuit, which consists of four resistors connected to the output of each PMT, as shown in Figure 3.9. This network produces four output signals, X^+, X^-, Y^+ and Y^- which are summed for all the PMTs. The relative magnitudes and signs of these summed signals then define the estimated (X,Y) location of the scintillation event in the crystal given by:

$$X = \frac{X^+ - X^-}{X^+ + X^-}, Y = \frac{Y^+ - Y^-}{Y^+ + Y^-}. \tag{3.15}$$

In more recent digital cameras, the currents for all the PMTs are stored and position estimation is performed using computer algorithms after all the data have been acquired. Corrections for non-uniform performance of each PMT can easily be built into the digital system.

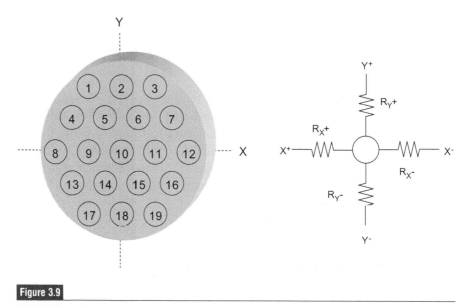

(left) Nineteen PMTs in a hexagonal arrangement on an NaI(Tl) crystal. (right) The four-resistor network attached to each PMT.

Pulse height analyzer

In addition to recording the individual components X^+, X^-, Y^+ and Y^-, the summed signal $\Sigma(X^++X^-+Y^++Y^-)$, termed the 'z-signal', is sent to a pulse-height analyzer (PHA). The role of the PHA is to determine which of the recorded events correspond to γ-rays that have not been scattered within tissue (primary radiation) and should be retained, and which have been Compton scattered in the patient, do not contain any useful spatial information, and so should be rejected. Since the amplitude of the voltage pulse from the PMT is proportional to the energy of the detected γ-ray, discriminating on the basis of the magnitude of the output of the PMT is equivalent to discriminating on the basis of γ-ray energy. A multiple-channel analyzer (MCA), in which the term 'channel' refers to a specific energy range, uses an analogue-to-digital converter to digitize the signal, and then to produce a pulse-height spectrum, i.e. a plot of the number of events from the PMTs as a function of the output voltage level. The number of channels in an MCA can be more than a thousand, allowing essentially a complete energy spectrum to be produced, as shown in Figure 3.10. After digitization, the upper and lower threshold values for accepting the γ-rays are applied.

At first sight it might seem that only a single threshold voltage equivalent to a 140 keV γ-ray which passes directly through tissue to the detector without scattering would suffice. However, γ-rays which have been scattered by only a very small angle still have useful information and so should be recorded. In addition, there are non-uniformities in the response of different parts of the NaI(Tl) crystal, and similarly with the PMTs, both of which will produce a range of output voltages

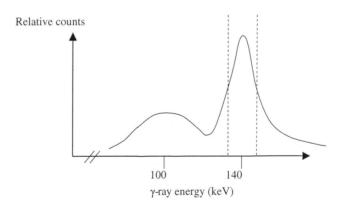

Figure 3.10

Readout from a multi-channel analyzer showing the number of counts recorded from a patient as a function of γ-ray energy. The dashed lines show the energy resolution of the camera, defined as the FWHM of the main photopeak centred at 140 keV.

even from mono-energetic γ-rays. Compton scattering of the γ-rays within the scintillation crystal itself also causes small and variable reductions in γ-ray energy. The energy resolution of the system is defined as the full-width-half-maximum (FWHM) of the photopeak, shown in Figure 3.10, and typically is about 14 keV (or 10%) for most gamma cameras without a patient present. The narrower the FWHM of the system the better it is at discriminating between unscattered and scattered γ-rays. In a clinical scan with the patient in place, the threshold level for accepting the 'photopeak' is set to a slightly larger value, typically 20%. For example, a 20% window around a 140 keV photopeak means that γ-rays with values of 127 to 153 keV are accepted.

3.6.4 Instrument dead time

If an injected dose of radiotracer is very large, the total number of γ-rays striking the scintillation crystal can exceed the recording capabilities of the system: this is particularly true at the beginning of a clinical scan when radioactivity is at its highest level. This limitation is due to the finite recovery and reset times required for various electronic circuits in the gamma camera. There are two types of behaviour exhibited by the system components, termed 'paralysable' and 'non-paralysable'. Paralysable behaviour is a phenomenon in which a component of the system cannot respond to a new event until a fixed time after the previous one, irrespective of whether that component is already in a non-responsive state. For example, each time a γ-ray strikes the scintillation crystal it produces an excited electronic state, which decays in 230 ns to release a number of photons. If another γ-ray strikes the same spot in the crystal before the excited state decays, then it will take a further 230 ns to decay, and only one set of photons will be produced even though two γ-rays have struck the crystal. A very high rate of γ-rays striking the detector, therefore, can potentially result in a considerably elongated dead-time. If the radioactivity level is very high, then this instrument 'dead time' becomes longer, and so the number of recorded events can actually decrease. In contrast, non-paralysable components cannot respond for a set time, irrespective of the level of radioactivity. For example, the Anger logic circuit and PHA take a certain time to process a given electrical input signal, and during this time any further events are simply not recorded: this time is fixed, and is not elongated if further scintillation events occur. Usually the overall 'dead-time' (τ) of the system is determined by the latter non-paralysable components, and is given by:

$$\tau = \frac{N - n}{nN},$$

(3.16)

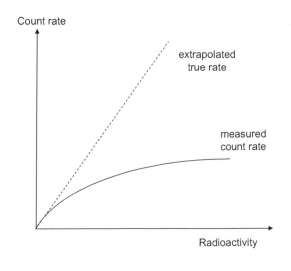

Count rate

extrapolated
true rate

measured
count rate

Radioactivity

Figure 3.11

Correction curve used to account for dead time losses. At very low count rates, the true rate and measured count rate are linearly related. As the radioactivity increases, the measured count rate reaches an asymptotic value, well below the true value.

where N is the true count rate (number of scintillations per second), and n is the measured count rate. The maximum measurable count rate is given by $1/\tau$.

Corrections for the dead-time are based upon calibrations using phantoms of known radioactivity, and also independent electronic measurements of the dead time of individual components of the system. For example, Figure 3.11 shows a plot of measured count rate vs radioactivity from a calibrated source showing the asymptotic behaviour described by Equation (3.16). Experimentally, this type of curve can be produced by imaging a source with known radioactivity, and acquiring images at different time points as the source radioactivity decays (data points on the right of the graph at high count rates are acquired at the beginning of this experiment). This gives a calibration curve for correcting the acquired images.

Example 3.3   Suppose that the true count rate in a gamma camera is 10 000 per second, but the measured rate is only 8000 per second. What is the dead time of the system?

Solution   From Equation (3.16) the value of τ is given as 25 μs. So rather than acquiring one count every 100 μs (the true value), there is a 25 μs effective delay and one event is recorded every 125 μs.

3.7 Image characteristics

Planar scintigraphy scans have no background signal since there is no natural γ-ray emission from the body, and therefore the images have a high intrinsic contrast. However, a large proportion of emitted γ-rays are scattered in the body and, if not removed, would result in a significant random background signal which would reduce the image contrast. Therefore quite severe collimation is required, which reduces the number of recorded events well below that of planar X-rays, for example, and therefore the SNR is much lower. Collimation also introduces significant depth-dependent broadening, Equation (3.13), and the requirement for low-pass filtering of the images due to the low SNR further degrades the spatial resolution.

Signal-to-noise

Since radioactive decay is a statistical process, in the sense that the spatial distribution of radioactivity at any one time does not have a single value but an average one with associated standard deviation according to the Poisson distribution (Section 2.8.1), the image SNR is proportional to the square root of the total number of detected γ-rays. This is exactly the same situation as for X-ray imaging. Factors that affect the SNR include:

(i) The amount of radiotracer administered, the time after administering the radiotracer at which imaging begins, the amount of radiotracer that accumulates in the organ being imaged, and the total time of the scan. Organs that are deep within the patient, or on the opposite side to the planar detector will experience more tissue attenuation of the γ-rays, and therefore lower SNR, than organs closer to the detector.

(ii) The intrinsic sensitivity of the gamma camera. Since parameters that affect the SNR such as the crystal thickness are fixed, the only factors that can be changed are the collimator properties (septal length, thickness and separation) and geometry (parallel, pinhole, converging or diverging).

(iii) Post-acquisition image filtering – due to the relatively low SNR of nuclear medicine images, a low-pass filter is often applied to the image (see Section 1.6). This filter increases the SNR but blurs the image, reducing the spatial resolution. The properties of the filter must be chosen carefully to maximize the CNR.

Spatial resolution

The spatial resolution of the image is given by the combination of two major instrument components:

$$R_{system} = \sqrt{R_{gamma}^2 + R_{coll}^2}, \tag{3.17}$$

where R_{gamma} is the intrinsic spatial resolution of the gamma camera and R_{coll} is determined by the collimator geometry. Contributions to R_{gamma} include the uncertainty in the exact location at which light is produced in the scintillation crystal, determined by the thickness of the crystal, and also the intrinsic resolution of the Anger position encoder (either analogue or digital). A typical value of R_{gamma} lies in the range 3–5 mm. The contribution from R_{coll} depends upon the collimator type and also the depth within the body of the organ in which the radiotracer accumulates, as seen in Equation (3.13). Typical values for the overall system spatial resolution are approximately 1–2 cm at large depths within the body, and 5–8 mm close to the collimator surface.

Contrast and contrast-to-noise

The theoretical image contrast is extremely high in nuclear medicine since there is no background signal from tissues in which the radiotracer has not distributed. However, the presence of Compton scattered γ-rays produces a random background signal, with more scatter close to regions in which the radiotracer concentrates. Factors affecting the spatial resolution also affect the contrast through the 'partial volume' effect, in which image blurring causes signal 'bleed' from small areas of high signal intensity to those where no radiotracer is present. The parameters for low pass filtering of the final image must be chosen carefully since there is a compromise between too strong a filter reducing the contrast due to image blur and too weak a filter not reducing the noise sufficiently.

3.8 Clinical applications of planar scintigraphy

Over the past 20 years, the role of nuclear medicine in the clinic has changed significantly. For example, previous brain scanning has largely been replaced by PET, CT and MRI, and ventilation/perfusion scans are now largely performed using multi-detector CT for evaluating pulmonary embolism. The major clinical application of planar scintigraphy is whole-body bone scanning which constitutes about 20% of all nuclear medicine scans. In addition, the thyroid, gastrointestinal tract, liver and kidneys are scanned using planar scintigraphy with specialized agents. For example, ^{99m}Tc can be attached to small particles of sulphur colloid, less than 100 nm diameter, which concentrate in healthy Kupffer cells in the liver, spleen and bone marrow. Pathological conditions such as cirrhosis of the liver result in diseased Kupffer cells which can no longer uptake the radiotracer, and therefore areas of low signal intensity, 'cold spots', are present in the image.

Bone scanning and tumour detection

Whole body scanning using ^{99m}Tc phosphonates such as hydroxymethylene-diphosphonate (HMDP, trade name Osteoscan) can be used to detect bone tumours, and also soft-tissue tumours which cause deformation and remodeling of bone structure. The mode of concentration of these agents in bone is thought to involve the affinity of diphosphonate for the metabolically active bone mineral hydroxyapatite, which exhibits increased metabolic turnover during bone growth. The usual response of bone to a tumour is to form new bone at the site of the tumour. For example, spinal tumours, which consist of metastatic lesions growing in the spinal marrow space, cause the bone structure of the spine to remodel. This results in local uptake of the radiotracer. Scanning starts 2–3 hours after injection of the radiotracer into a patient's bloodstream to allow accumulation within the skeletal structure, and several scans with longitudinal overlap are used to cover the whole body, as shown in Figure 3.12. If any suspected tumours are detected, then further localized scans can be acquired. Bone infarctions or aggressive bone metastases often show up as signal voids in the nuclear medicine scan, since bone necrosis has occurred and there is no blood flow to deliver the radiotracer to that region.

Other radiotracers which can be used in tumour detection are ^{67}Ga-citrate and ^{201}Tl. Radiotracer ligands can also be designed for active targetting of specific tumours which are known to express certain receptors. For example, ^{111}In-DTPA-octreotide has been designed to target tumours which over-express somatostatin receptors.

3.9 Single photon emission computed tomography (SPECT)

SPECT uses two or three gamma cameras which rotate around the patient detecting γ-rays at a number of different angles. Either filtered backprojection or iterative techniques are used to reconstruct multiple two-dimensional axial slices from the acquired projections. The relationship between planar scintigraphy and SPECT is analogous to that between planar X-ray imaging and CT. SPECT uses essentially the same instrumentation and many of the same radiotracers as planar scintigraphy, and most SPECT machines can also be used for planar scans. The majority of SPECT scans are used for myocardial perfusion studies to detect coronary artery disease or myocardial infarction, although SPECT is also used for brain studies to detect areas of reduced blood flow associated with stroke, epilepsy or neurodegenerative diseases such as Alzheimers.

Since the array of PMTs is two-dimensional in nature, the data can be reconstructed as a series of adjacent slices, as shown in Figure 3.13. A 360° rotation is

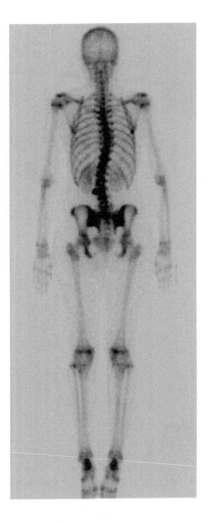

Figure 3.12

A whole-body scan, made from a composite of ten different scans, showing the uptake of ^{99m}Tc-methylenediphosphonate within the body. The faint background is due to Compton-scattered γ-rays.

generally needed in SPECT since the source-to-detector distance affects the distribution of γ-ray scatter in the body, the degree of tissue attenuation and also the spatial resolution, and so projections acquired at 180° to one another are not identical. A converging collimator is often used in SPECT to increase the SNR of the scan. In a SPECT brain scan each image of a multi-slice data set is formed from typically 500 000 counts, with a spatial resolution of ~7 mm. Myocardial SPECT has a lower number of counts, typically 100 000 per image, and a spatial resolution about twice as coarse as that of the brain scan (since the source to detector distance is much larger due to the size of the body).

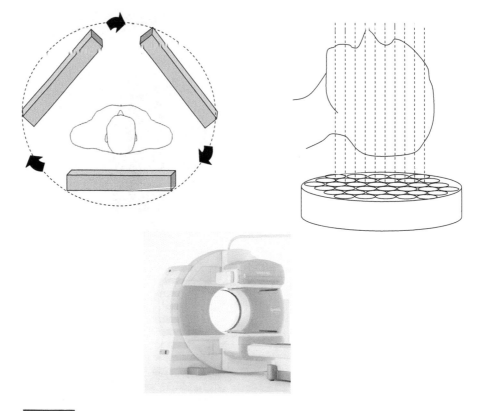

(top left) A three-head rotating gamma camera SPECT system for imaging the torso. (top right) Multiple 2D slices can be acquired in the longitudinal direction. (bottom) A 2-head SPECT camera: the heads can be moved inwards to image the brain, or outwards for the body.

3.10   Data processing in SPECT

Before the process of image reconstruction, the data must be corrected for a number of instrument variabilities, as well as intrinsic factors such as scatter and depth-dependent attenuation.

3.10.1   Scatter correction

A feature of SPECT imaging is that it is able to acquire fully quantitative images in which the image intensity can be related to an absolute concentration of radiotracer for detailed pharmacokinetic analysis, if needed. However, fully quantitative assessment requires accurate correction of image intensities. The first step in data processing is scatter correction. Since the accepted range of energies for the ^{99m}Tc photopeak is 127–153 keV (an energy resolution of 20%), it is easy to calculate that a 140 keV γ-ray that has been Compton scattered by a very large angle, up to 50°, is also detected within this energy window. The contribution from scattered γ-rays is typically of the same order as those which have not been scattered, even with the lead collimator in place. The number of scattered γ-rays is greatest closest to areas in which there is a high concentration of radiotracer, and so a position dependent scatter correction is required. The most common method uses a dual-energy, or multiple-energy, window and a multi-channel analyzer. The primary window is centred at the photopeak, with a second 'subwindow' set to a lower energy range, for example 92–125 keV, as shown in Figure 3.14. The primary window contains contributions from both scattered and unscattered γ-rays, but the subwindow should have contributions only from scattered γ-rays. Data projections are now formed from the primary and secondary windows separately, and the scatter projections are scaled by a scaling factor before being subtracted from the primary projections. The scaling factor is given by $W_m/2W_s$, where W_m is the width of the primary window (26 keV) and W_s that of the secondary window (33 keV): the factor of 2 in the denominator is one that has been determined empirically. A triple-energy window (TEW) approach can also be used, in which the main photopeak typically has a width of 15% centred at 140 keV and the two subwindows are very narrow, each 3 keV wide centred at 126 and 153 keV, respectively. This is also shown in Figure 3.14. The data processing procedure is to divide the counts in each pixel of the scatter projections by the width in keV of the scatter window, add the two scatter window projections together, multiply the

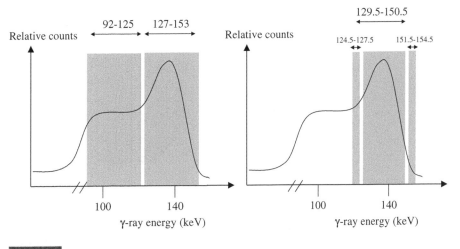

Figure 3.14

Two methods of scatter correction for SPECT. (left) A dual-energy window approach, and (right) a triple-energy window approach.

resultant projections by half of the photopeak window width in keV, and finally subtract the result from the original projections.

3.10.2 Attenuation correction

Since γ-rays from radiotracers located in the centre of the patient have to pass through more tissue to reach the detector than those present in organs much closer to the surface, the γ-rays from deeper within the body are attenuated more. Therefore, some form of attenuation correction is required for accurate quantitation. Attenuation correction can be performed using one of two methods. The first, known as Chang's multiplicative method, assumes that the tissue attenuation coefficient is uniform throughout the part of the body being imaged. An initial image is formed by filtered backprojection without any corrections, and this image is used to estimate the outline of the body part being imaged and therefore the distance (x) that the γ-rays have to travel through tissue to the detector. Each projection can then be scaled up by an appropriate factor given by $e^{+\mu x}$. A schematic example of this process is shown in Figure 3.15. The assumption of a uniform attenuation coefficient works reasonably well for the brain and abdomen, but cannot be used for cardiac or thoracic imaging in which tissue attenuation is highly spatially dependent.

The second technique uses a transmission scan, usually acquired simultaneously with the actual patient scan, with a source containing radioactive gadolinium (^{153}Gd) which emits γ-rays with an energy of ~102 keV. The half-life of ^{153}Gd is 242 days and so the radioactivity can be assumed to be constant over several

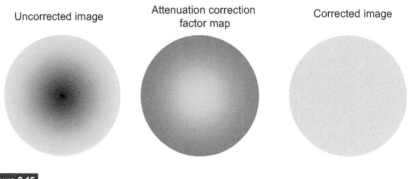

| Uncorrected image | Attenuation correction factor map | Corrected image |

Figure 3.15

Demonstration of Chang's multiplicative method for attenuation correction. (left) An uncorrected SPECT image of a sphere which is filled with a material with uniform radioactivity. The dark area in the middle occurs since γ-rays are attenuated as they pass through the material. (middle) Based upon the outline of the phantom, a correction factor map is produced, with a high scaling factor at the centre and lower scaling factor to the outside. (right) Application of the correction factor gives an image which reflects much more accurately the uniform distribution of radiotracer.

months. Since the energy of the Gd is much lower than that of the ^{99m}Tc γ-rays, dual energy windows can be used to acquire both ^{153}Gd and ^{99m}Tc data at the same time. Clearly there will be some 'bleedthrough' from scattered γ-rays from ^{99m}Tc to the ^{153}Gd window, but this can be corrected by using a third window in-between the other two and using methods described previously for scatter correction. By comparing the signal intensities of each ^{153}Gd projection taken with the patient in place with reference scans acquired without the patient, the attenuation coefficient at each position can be calculated and the image of the patient corrected.

3.10.3 Image reconstruction

Two methods can be chosen to reconstruct SPECT images, either filtered backprojection or iterative methods, the latter of which are increasingly being used as computational power increases. Filtered backprojection algorithms are essentially identical to those described previously for CT, and so are not described further here.

The general scheme for iterative reconstruction is shown in Figure 3.16. It starts with an initial image estimate, which can be a very simple geometric shape. The forward projection step computes projections from the estimated image, and

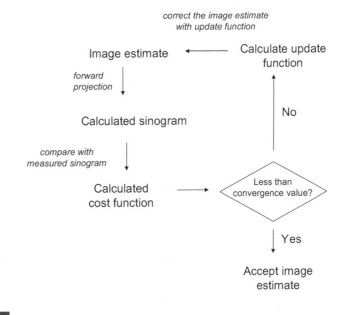

Figure 3.16

An iterative reconstruction algorithm for SPECT. The algorithm loops around until the calculated cost function falls below a pre-defined threshold value.

assembles them into a sinogram. During this process, estimates of the distribution of scattered γ-rays, spatially-dependent attenuation and a depth-dependent point spread function can be built into the forward model. The sinogram is then compared with the one that is actually acquired, and the difference between the two is calculated as a cost function. This cost function can be a simple sum-of-squares difference between the actual and predicted data on a pixel-by-pixel basis, or can weight more heavily the areas of the sinogram which have the highest signal intensity. Based upon the cost function the estimated data are now updated to improve the similarity between actual and estimated data. There are a number of possible update functions, and the appropriate choice is an active area of mathematical development. Since there is never perfect agreement between the measured and estimated sinograms, a lower threshold value of the cost function, which is determined to be acceptable, is defined (alternatively the total number of iterations can be given a maximum value). At each stage of the iteration, this calculated cost function is compared with this threshold. If it is above the threshold, i.e. the reconstruction is not 'good enough', then the estimated image is recalculated using an update function based upon the error. Iterative reconstruction is a very computationally intensive process, and there are a number of methods that have been devised to speed it up. One general class is termed 'ordered subsets', in which the early iterative stages use only a small subset of the acquired profiles, with this number increasing to the full amount as the iteration progresses. The most common algorithm used is referred to as the maximum-likelihood expectation-maximum (ML-EM) method.

3.11   SPECT/CT

Since 2005 there has been an increasing trend to combine SPECT with CT in a combined scanner [2;3]. In 2008 there were approximately 1000 SPECT/CT systems installed worldwide. A SPECT/CT system acquires data from the two image modalities with a single integrated patient bed and gantry. The two imaging studies are performed with the patient remaining on the table, which is moved from the CT scanner to the SPECT system, as shown in Figure 3.17. Typical clinical systems use a two-head SPECT camera with a multi-slice CT scanner. The primary advantages of a combined SPECT/CT over a stand-alone SPECT system are: (i) improved attenuation correction for SPECT reconstruction using the high resolution anatomical information from the CT scanner, and (ii) the fusion of high-resolution anatomical (CT) with functional (SPECT) information, allowing the anatomical location of radioactive 'hot' or 'cold' spots to be defined much better with reduced partial volume effects compared to SPECT alone. In terms of the advantages of CT-based

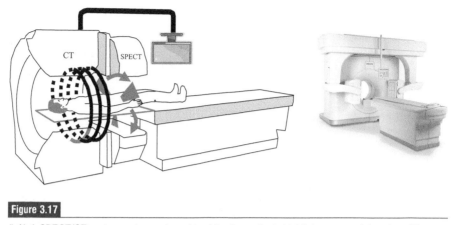

Figure 3.17

(left) A SPECT/CT system using a shared bed for the patient. (right) A commercial system. There are two gamma cameras, one above and one below the patient, and a circular entry for the multi-detector CT.

attenuation correction vs. ^{153}Gd transmission scans, the CT data have a far higher SNR, they can be acquired much more quickly, there is no cross-talk between X-rays and γ-rays, and the CT source has a constant flux over time whereas the ^{153}Gd source decays slowly. The only disadvantage is that the scans are acquired serially rather than simultaneously, which can potentially lead to misregistrations between SPECT data and the CT-derived attenuation maps if the patient moves position.

3.12   Clinical applications of SPECT and SPECT/CT

As outlined earlier, the major application of SPECT is to cardiac studies. Given this focus, specialized instrumentation specifically for rapid cardiac scanning is being introduced, as covered later in this section.

3.12.1   Myocardial perfusion

The most important application of SPECT is for assessing myocardial perfusion to diagnose coronary artery disease (CAD) and damage to the heart muscle following an infarction (a heart attack). CAD is one of the major causes of death in the western world. Atherosclerosis can cause hardening and narrowing of the coronary arteries, or else atherosclerotic plaques can build up within the artery wall, causing clots and a reduction in the blood flow to heart muscle. Patients with known high risk factors or who have chest pain and/or abnormal EKG recordings often are referred for a 'nuclear cardiac stress test'. The most common agent used in these

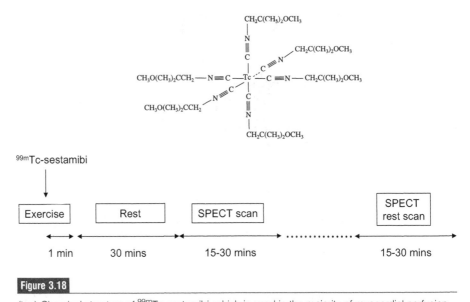

Figure 3.18

(top) Chemical structure of ^{99m}Tc-sestamibi, which is used in the majority of myocardial perfusion scans. (bottom) The scanning protocol for the nuclear medicine cardiac stress test.

studies is ^{99m}Tc-sestamibi (trade name cardiolite), the structure of which is shown in Figure 3.18. Since this compound has a positive charge, it accumulates in the mitochondria in heart muscle. The organic side-chains of the molecule are designed so that the complex is of intermediate lipophilicity. Although other agents such as ^{201}Tl can also be used for these tests, ^{99m}Tc is increasingly being used primarily due to a lower administered radioactive dose.

Figure 3.18 shows a block diagram of the protocol for the stress test. The first stage involves injecting a relatively low dose, ~8 mCi, of radiotracer while the patient is exercising on a stationary bicycle or treadmill. Exercise continues for about a minute after injection to ensure clearance of the tracer from the blood. Uptake of the radiotracer is proportional to local blood flow, with about 5% of the dose going to the heart. Exercise increases the oxygen demand of the heart causing normal coronary arteries to dilate, with blood flow increasing to a value typically three to five times greater than that at rest, with uniform uptake of the radiotracer within the left ventricular myocardium. If the coronary arteries are blocked, however, they cannot dilate and so the blood flow cannot increase sufficiently to satisfy the oxygen demand of the heart, and this shows up as an area of low signal intensity on the SPECT scan. The results of this first SPECT scan are compared with one acquired at rest, which is typically acquired much later in the day. Figure 3.19 shows a series of short-axis slices from a myocardial SPECT scan, along with a schematic of the heart which shows the orientation of the images. The multi-slice data can be reconstructed and displayed as oblique-, long- or short-axis

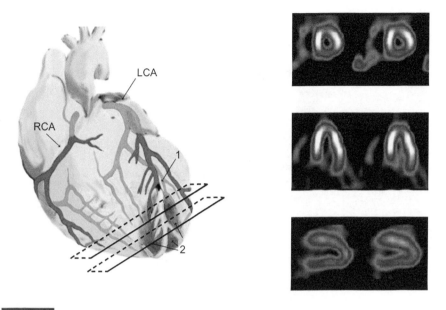

Figure 3.19

(left) Structure of the heart showing the right coronary artery (RCA) and left coronary artery (LCA). Arrow 1 shows one common site of vessel occlusion, whereas the areas (2) indicated by the small arrows are often associated with myocardial infarction. (right) The top row shows SPECT scans acquired in the planes indicated on the schematic of the heart. The acquired data can be reformatted to be shown in any direction, as shown in the two lower sets of images which represent two planes orthogonal to that in the top row.

views of the heart, greatly aiding diagnosis. A cardiac SPECT system typically has only two rotating gamma cameras, with the detectors oriented at $90°$ to one another. Only a $180°$ rotation is used to form the image since the heart is positioned close to the front of the thorax and well to the left of the body.

A SPECT myocardial perfusion protocol can take up to $2\frac{1}{2}$ hours of procedure time, including half-an-hour for scanning. Since this type of perfusion scan is so prevalent, a few specialized cardiac SPECT systems have been designed to reduce this imaging time significantly, and also to improve the spatial resolution of the scans. One approach, called dSPECT (dynamic SPECT) uses a detector placed over and to one side of the chest with nine solid state cadmium zinc telluride (CZT) detectors rather than the conventional NaI(Tl) crystal. CZT has significantly better energy resolution than NaI(Tl) and also a higher attenuation coefficient, although it cannot be made into detectors as thick as a NaI(Tl) crystal. The set-up, shown in Figure 3.20, also allows the patient to sit up rather than lie down, which reduces patient motion. A second set-up, termed a CardiArc system, uses the same solid state CZT detectors (although NaI(Tl) can also be used), but has a very large semi-circular array of these detectors, each of which are ~2.5 mm in size. All of the signal

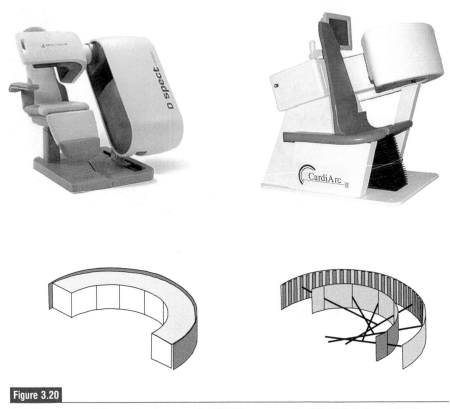

Figure 3.20

(top) Two commercial specialized myocardial SPECT scanners, the DSPECT (left) and CardiArc (right). (bottom) Showing the mode of operation of the CardiArc scanner using a six-slit horizontal collimator which is in constant motion, and the lead vanes used for vertical collimation.

processing hardware is attached directly to a circuit board, with the detectors on the other side of the circuit board. For collimation a thin sheet of lead is placed between the patient and the detectors with only six thin slots in the vertical direction. Back-and-forth movement of this collimator by up to ~25 cm enables scanning through the patient with a very fine angular increment of ~0.14° (compared to 3° for conventional SPECT). For vertical collimation, thin lead 'vanes' are used to separate the different levels of CZT detectors, which enables multi-slice images to be acquired. Again, the patient can be scanned in a more natural sitting position. Myocardial scan time reduction to 2–4 minutes is possible with either of these relatively new systems.

3.12.2 Brain SPECT and SPECT/CT

SPECT studies are also performed to measure blood perfusion in the brain, most commonly using ^{99m}Tc-exametazime (trade name Ceretec), a neutral complex which

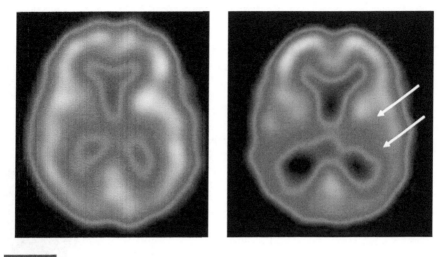

Figure 3.21

(left) Brain SPECT from a healthy patient. (right) Corresponding scan from a patient with Alzheimer's disease. The arrows point to significantly reduced activity in the temporal and parietal lobes.

passes through the blood brain barrier due to its low molecular weight, relative lipophilicity, and zero charge. The agent is metabolized inside the cells into a more hydrophilic species which cannot easily diffuse back out of the cell and therefore accumulates over time to an amount proportional to the regional cerebral blood flow (rCBF). Uptake in the brain reaches a maximum of ~5% of the injected dose within one minute of injection. Up to 15% of the activity is eliminated from the brain within two minutes post-injection, after which the concentration of the radio-tracer remains constant for the next 24 hours. A healthy brain has symmetric blood perfusion patterns in both hemispheres, with higher blood flow in grey matter than white matter. Diseases which cause altered perfusion patterns include epilepsy, cerebral infarction, schizophrenia and dementia. One commonly studied form of dementia is Alzheimer's disease, which is characterized by bilateral decreased flow in the temporal and parietal lobes with normal flow in the primary sensorimotor and visual cortices, as shown in Figure 3.21. Stroke patients often show signifi-cantly reduced blood perfusion on the side of the brain in which the stroke has occurred.

3.13 Positron emission tomography (PET)

Similar to SPECT, PET is a tomographic technique which also uses radiotracers [4;5]. However, PET has between 100 and 1000 times higher SNR as well as significantly better spatial resolution than SPECT (6). The fundamental difference

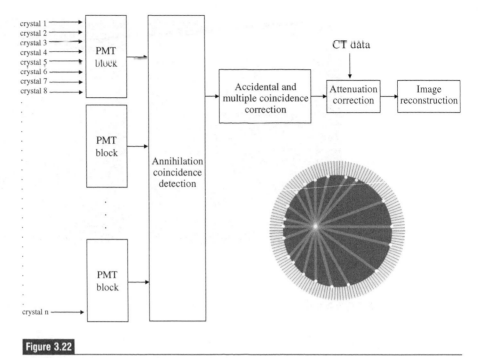

(top) The elements of a PET/CT system. (inset) Formation of lines-of-response in the PET detector ring.

between the two imaging techniques is that the radiotracers used in PET emit positrons which, after annihilation with an electron in tissue, result in the formation of *two* γ-rays with energies of 511 keV each. These two γ-rays have trajectories 180° apart and strike solid-state detectors which are positioned in a series of complete rings around the patient. This forms an intrinsic line-of-reconstruction (LOR) without the need for any collimation, as shown in Figure 3.22. The much higher SNR of PET compared to SPECT arises from several factors including: (i) collimation not being required, (ii) reduced attenuation of higher energy (511 keV vs. 140 keV) γ-rays in tissue, and (iii) the use of a complete ring of detectors. In the past five years, stand-alone PET scanners have largely been replaced with hybrid PET/CT scanners which use a single patient bed to slide between the two systems [7]. The rationale for the hybrid system is similar to that for SPECT/CT, namely improved attenuation correction and the ability to fuse morphological and functional information. A photograph of a commercial PET/CT system is shown later in the chapter in Figure 3.27.

A general block diagram of the instrumentation for PET is shown in Figure 3.22. The detectors (typically many thousands) consist of small crystals of bismuth germanate (BGO), which are coupled to PMTs: the resulting output voltages are then digitized. After correction of the acquired data for accidental coincidences and attenuation effects using the CT images, the PET image is reconstructed using either filtered backprojection or iterative methods. The most recent technical innovation in commercial PET/CT scanners is time-of-flight (TOF) technology, in which the SNR is improved by very accurate measurement of the exact time at which each γ-ray hits the detector. This allows localization within the LOR, and is discussed in detail in Section 3.20.

PET/CT has its major clinical applications in the general areas of oncology, cardiology and neurology. In oncology, whole body imaging is used to identify both primary tumours and secondary metastatic disease remote from the primary source. The major disadvantages of PET/CT are the requirement for an on-site cyclotron to produce positron emitting radiotracers, and the high associated costs.

3.14 Radiotracers used for PET/CT

Isotopes such as ^{11}C, ^{15}O, ^{18}F and ^{13}N used in PET/CT undergo radioactive decay by emitting a positron, i.e. a positively charged electron (e^+), and a neutrino:

$$^{18}_{9}F \rightarrow {}^{18}_{8}O + e^+ + \text{neutrino}$$

$$^{11}_{6}C \rightarrow {}^{11}_{5}B + e^+ + \text{neutrino}.$$

The positron travels a short distance (an average of 0.1–2 mm depending upon the particular radiotracer) in tissue before annihilating with an electron. This annihilation results in the formation of two γ-rays, each with an energy of 511 keV. Table 3.2 lists commonly used PET radiotracers with their applications and half-lives.

Radiotracers for PET must be synthesized on-site using a cyclotron, and are structural analogues of biologically active molecules in which one or more of the atoms have been replaced by a radioactive atom. Therefore, after production of the

Table 3.2: Properties and applications of the most common PET radiotracers

Radionuclide	Half-life (minutes)	Radiotracer	Clinical applications
^{18}F	109.7	^{18}FDG	oncology, inflammation, cardiac viability
^{11}C	20.4	^{11}C-palmitate	cardiac metabolism
^{15}O	2.07	$H_2{}^{15}O$	cerebral blood flow
^{13}N	9.96	$^{13}NH_3$	cardiac blood flow
^{82}Rb	1.27	$^{82}RbCl_2$	cardiac perfusion

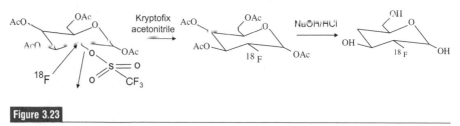

Figure 3.23

The most common synthesis of ^{18}FDG.

particular radionuclide it must be incorporated, via rapid chemical synthesis, into the corresponding radiotracer. For speed and safety these syntheses are carried out robotically. Such robotic units are available commercially to synthesize, for example, ^{18}F-fluorodeoxyglucose (FDG), $^{15}O_2$, $C^{15}O_2$, $C^{15}O$, $^{13}NH_3$ and $H_2{}^{15}O$. The most common radiotracer, used in 80% of studies, is FDG, the structure of which is shown in Figure 3.23, which also illustrates its basic synthesis [8]. Once injected into the bloodstream, FDG is actively transported across the blood/brain barrier into cells. Inside the cell, FDG is phosphorylated by glucose hexokinase to give FDG-6-phosphate. This chemical is trapped inside the cell, since it cannot react with G-6-phosphate dehydrogenase, which is the next step in the glycolytic cycle, because the hydroxyl group at the 2-carbon is a requirement for the process. Since a high glucose metabolic rate is characteristic of many types of tumour, these show up as hot spots in oncological PET scans.

The only PET radiotracer that can be produced from an on-site generator rather than a cyclotron is ^{82}Rb. The process uses ^{82}Sr as the parent isotope, which has a half life of 600 hours. The physical set-up is quite similar to the technetium generator described in Section 3.4, with the ^{82}Sr adsorbed on stannic oxide in a lead-shielded column. The column is eluted with NaCl solution, and the eluent is in the form of rubidium chloride which is injected intravenously. The ^{82}Rb rapidly clears from the bloodstream and is extracted by myocardial tissue in a manner analogous to potassium. Since the half-life of ^{82}Rb is just over one minute, scans have to be acquired relatively quickly using a very high initial dose of ~50 mCi. Areas of myocardial infarction are visualized within two to seven minutes post-injection as cold areas on the myocardial scan. The spatial resolution of ^{82}Rb images is slightly lower than for other radiotracers since the positron emitted has a higher energy and therefore travels further before annihilation.

3.15   Instrumentation for PET/CT

The instrumentation in the PET section of a PET/CT scanner is significantly different from a SPECT scanner, with many thousands of small solid-state detectors, and additional annihilation coincidence circuitry. However, there are also several components which are very similar to SPECT systems, including multi-channel pulse height analyzers and photomultiplier tubes.

3.15.1 Scintillation crystals

Although NaI(Tl) crystals can be used for PET, the material has a low detection efficiency at 511 keV, meaning that the crystal would have to be very thick for high SNR and this would result in poor spatial resolution. The properties of various materials which are used as scintillation crystal detectors in PET are shown in Table 3.3 [9]. The ideal detector crystal has:

(a) a high γ-ray detection efficiency,
(b) a short decay time to allow a short coincidence resolving time to be used, (Section 3.16.2),
(c) a high emission intensity (the number of photons per detected γ-ray) to allow more crystals to be coupled to a single PMT, reducing the complexity and cost of the PET scanner,
(d) an emission wavelength near 400 nm which corresponds to the maximum sensitivity for standard PMTs,
(e) optical transparency at the emission wavelength, and
(f) an index of refraction close to 1.5 to ensure efficient transmission of light between the crystal and the PMT.

Bismuth germanate detectors are used in the majority of commercial PET/CT systems, as BGO has a high density and effective atomic number giving it a high

Table 3.3: Properties of PET detectors

	Decay time (ns)	Emission intensity	Efficiency (ϵ^2)	$\lambda_{emitted}$ (nm)	η
BGO	300	0.15	0.72	480	2.15
LSO(Ce)	40	0.75	0.69	420	1.82
BaF$_2$	0.8$_{prim}$, 600$_{sec}$	0.12	0.34	220, 310	1.49
GSO(Ce)	60$_{prim}$, 600$_{sec}$	0.3	0.57	430	1.85
NaI(Tl)	230$_{prim}$, 10$^4_{sec}$	1.0	0.24	410	1.85

GSO(Ce):cerium-doped gadolinium orthosilicate (Gd$_2$SiO$_5$),LSO(Ce): cerium-doped lutetium orthosilicate (Lu$_2$SiO$_5$). Both primary and secondary decay times are reported, efficiency values are for 2 cm thickness crystals and represent detection of both γ-rays striking the two detectors, η is the refractive index, and decay times are expressed as primary and secondary decays; the intensity is relative to a value of 1.0 for NaI(Tl).

linear attenuation coefficient and hence high efficiency. The major disadvantage of BGO is its low emission intensity, meaning that a maximum of 16 crystal elements can be coupled to each PMT. An alternative material, LSO(Ce), has a much higher intensity and almost as high an efficiency, and is currently being commercially integrated into newer systems, particularly time-of-flight (TOF) scanners for which its very short decay time is highly advantageous. A third material, GSO(Ce), is also used in some PET/CT systems. BaF_2 has the shortest decay time, but has not yet found widespread commercial utility.

Detection of the anti-parallel γ-rays uses a large number of scintillation crystals which are placed in a circular ring surrounding the patient. Coupling each crystal to a single PMT would give the highest possible spatial resolution but would also increase the cost prohibitively. Modern PET scanners are based upon a 'block detector' design, which consists of a large block of BGO (dimensions ~50 × 50 × 30 mm) which has a series of partial cuts through it, with the cuts filled with light-reflecting material, as shown in Figure 3.24. The cuts prevent light which is formed at the top of the crystal from producing a very broad light spread function by the time the photon has passed through the entire 30 mm depth. An eight-by-eight array of partial cuts is produced, and each block can be considered to contain effectively 64 separate detectors, each with dimensions ~6 × 6 mm with a depth of 30 mm. Four PMTs are coupled to each BGO block and localization of the detected γ-ray to a particular crystal is performed using exactly the same Anger principle as outlined in Section 3.6.3. The dimensions of the cuts in the block are designed to provide a linear output to each PMT, performing the same task as the resistor network in the gamma camera. A modification to this scheme is termed quadrant sharing, shown also in Figure 3.24, in which larger PMTs are used and

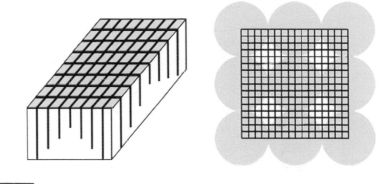

Figure 3.24

(left) A large BGO crystal cut into 64 effective separate elements. The partial cuts are filled with light-reflecting material. (right) Quadrant-sharing arrangement of the BGO crystals with PMTs shown by the circles.

positioned so that they each overlap approximately one quarter of four adjacent blocks. This reduces further the number of PMTs required.

A full PET ring is made up of many of these blocks, with several thousand individual detectors. Typical ring diameters are either 70 or 85 cm for abdominal scanners, or ~45 cm for head scanners. A number of these rings are stacked axially (in the patient head/foot direction) allowing a head/foot imaging field-of-view of ~16 cm. The dimensions of the individual elements in each block are important since they affect the overall spatial resolution of the PET system. The contribution from the detector size is approximately half the dimension of the detector, so ~2–3 mm for most PET systems.

3.15.2 Photomultiplier tubes and pulse height analyzer

The operation of these devices is essentially identical to that described previously for planar nuclear medicine and SPECT. When a γ-ray hits a BGO or LSO(Ce) detector crystal it produces a number of photons. These photons are converted into an amplified electrical signal, at the output of the PMT, which is fed into a multi-channel analyzer. If the voltage is within a pre-determined range, then the PHA generates a 'logic pulse', which is sent to the coincidence detector: typically, this logic pulse is 6–10 ns long. The energy resolution of BGO crystals is ~20%, so the energy window set for acceptance is typically 450–650 keV.

3.15.3 Annihilation coincidence detection

Each time that a signal is recorded in a given PET detector crystal it is given a 'time-stamp', with a precision typically between 1 and 2 ns. Since the two γ-rays from a positron annihilation event may originate from an area in the patient which is much closer to one side of the detector ring than the other, there is a difference in the arrival time of the two γ-rays at the respective detectors after the annihilation event, as shown on the left of Figure 3.25. A fixed 'coincidence resolving time' exists for the system, defined as the time-window that is allowed after the first γ-ray has been detected for a second γ-ray to be recorded and assigned to the same annihilation. Provided that this second γ-ray strikes a detector which is operated in coincidence with the first detector, then this pair of γ-rays is accepted as a 'true coincidence' and an LOR can be drawn between the two detectors. This process is called annihilation coincidence detection (ACD), and the steps involved are shown in in Figure 3.25. The first γ-ray from the annihilation strikes detector number 2 and a logic pulse is sent to the ACD circuit. Only those detectors numbered

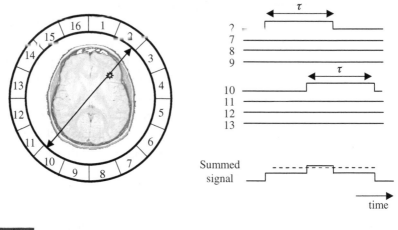

The principle of annihilation coincidence detection. (left) The two γ-rays reach detectors 2 and 10, triggering respective logic pulses of length τ. (right) If both logic pulses are sent to the coincidence detector within the system coincidence resolving time 2τ, then the summed signal lies above the threshold value (dashed line) and a coincidence is recorded.

between 7 and 13 are 'in coincidence' with detector number 2 since unscattered γ-rays which originate from within the head must lie within the volume defined by detectors 7–13, as shown in Figure 3.25. When the second γ-ray is detected in crystal 10 a second logic pulse is sent to the ACD circuit, which adds the two pulses together. If the summed signal is greater than a threshold set to a value just less than twice the amplitude of each individual logic pulse, then a coincidence is accepted and an LOR established between the two detectors. The coincidence resolving time is defined as twice the length of each logic pulse, with a value typically between 6 and 12 ns.

Example 3.4   Assume that the head is an ellipse with major dimensions 28 and 22 cm. The patient is placed within a head PET scanner with a circular arrangement, diameter 45 cm, of BGO detectors. What is the maximum time difference that can occur for an event between two detectors?

Solution   The maximum difference clearly corresponds to a scintillation event occurring either right at the front or at the back of the head. Assuming that the head is perfectly centred in the PET scanner, there is a 28 cm difference in the trajectories of the two γ-rays. Assuming that the γ-rays travel through tissue at the speed of light, 3×10^8 m/s, then the times of detection will be ~930 ps, or just less than 1 ns apart.

3.16 Two-dimensional and three-dimensional PET imaging

Commercial PET systems have a number of detector rings, up to 48 in total, which are stacked along the patient head/foot direction. Data can be acquired either in 2D multi-slice or full 3D mode, with the great majority of scans now acquired in 3D mode. The scanner has retractable lead collimation septa positioned between each ring: these septa are extended for 2D multi-slice operation and retracted for imaging in 3D mode. In 2D mode this collimation reduces the amount of scattered γ-rays detected and also has the characteristic of producing a uniform sensitivity profile along the axial dimension. This means that for whole body PET scans, in which the table has to be moved several times to cover the entire body length, the required overlap between successive table positions need only be ~1–2 cm. Image planes can be formed between two crystals in the same ring (direct planes), and also from crystals in adjacent rings (cross planes). For a system with n rings, there are n direct planes and n-1 cross planes, making a total of 2n-1 image planes, as shown in Figure 3.26.

Three-dimensional PET has a much higher sensitivity than 2D PET by about a factor of 10, primarily due to the elimination of the collimators. Given that the SNR is proportional to the square root of the number of counts recorded, this is equivalent to a scan time reduction of two orders of magnitude. However, without the collimators there are many more random coincidences and a far greater contribution from scattered γ-rays in 3D mode. In addition, the sensitivity profile in the axial direction is much higher at the centre of the scanner than at either end, and

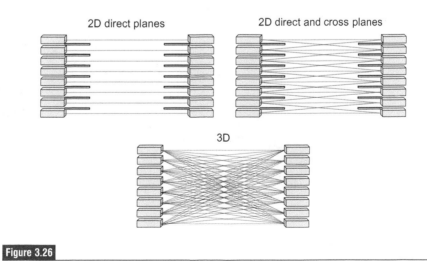

Figure 3.26

Three different data acquisition modes used for PET scans. Note that the septal collimators are retracted for 3D mode.

therefore for whole body scanning the overlap between table positions can be as high as 50% meaning that more positions are required. Nevertheless, the majority of studies are performed in 3D mode due to the far superior SNR.

3.17   PET/CT

Since 2006 no stand-alone commercial PET scanners have been produced, all are now integrated PET/CT systems. The reasons for combining PET and CT in a hybrid imaging system are essentially identical to those already outlined for SPECT/CT. The improved accuracy in attenuation correction and image fusion of morphological and functional data are particularly important in oncological studies which form the major applications of PET/CT. Studies which previously took up to an hour now typically take half the time since a separate PET calibration scan for attenuation correction is not necessary, and the CT calibration scan is extremely rapid. There are now well over 2000 PET/CT systems installed in the world. The hybrid system contains two separate detector rings and a common patient bed which slides between the two, as shown in Figure 3.27. Most PET/CT scanners have a 70 cm bore for both CT and PET. The very latest PET/CT scanners have a bore of 85 cm for larger patients, although the spatial resolution is somewhat degraded due to the larger ring size.

The major issue with PET/CT, as for SPECT/CT, is the mismatch between the data acquisition times of the two modalities. In the thorax and abdomen, MSCT acquires entire data sets in 1s or less, whereas the PET data are acquired over

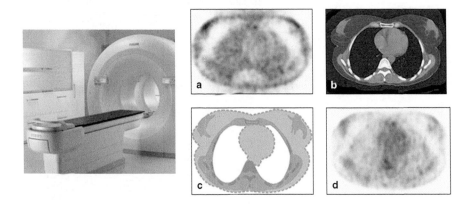

Figure 3.27

(left) A PET/CT scanner with two separate rings of detectors. A common bed slides the patient through the two scanners. (right) (a) An uncorrected PET, (b) a CT image, (c) the CT-derived attenuation map after segmentation of the CT image, and (d) the attenuation-corrected PET scan.

several minutes or more. Therefore, there can be a misregistration between the position of, for example a tumour in the CT and PET scans if there is significant displacement due to cardiac- or breathing-related patient motion. Currently, the very basic approach of blurring the CT data to match the PET images is used, but more sophisticated algorithms are under development. Figure 3.27 shows an example of a thoracic study using PET/CT, with attenuation correction from the high resolution CT data.

3.18 Data processing in PET/CT

Image reconstruction in PET is essentially identical to that in SPECT with both iterative algorithms and those based on filtered backprojection being used to form the image from all of the acquired LORs. Prior to image reconstruction, the data must be corrected for attenuation effects as well as for accidental and multiple coincidences, dead-time losses and scattered radiation.

3.18.1 Attenuation correction

Correction for attenuation effects in the patient is required for PET for the same reasons as for SPECT. Prior to the advent of combined PET/CT scanners, a transmission-based calibration using ^{68}Ge was used to estimate the required attenuation, in direct analogy to the ^{153}Gd source in SPECT. This procedure has been replaced by the PET/CT scanner, since the SNR and spatial resolution of the CT-based attenuation data are far superior to that of the PET calibration method, and much faster to acquire. After acquisition of the calibration scan the CT images are segmented into a number of different tissue types (muscle, lipid, bone) to which standard values of μ at 511 keV are assigned. Since the spatial resolution of the attenuation map is much finer than that of the PET scan, the CT-based attenuation map is smoothed to match the resolution of the PET scan before implementing the attenuation correction. This spatial smoothing is also important for abdominal imaging, in which the CT data represents a snapshot, i.e. the abdomen in only one position during the respiratory and cardiac cycles, whereas the PET scan is acquired over many minutes and therefore represents a time-average.

3.18.2 Corrections for accidental and multiple coincidences

Accidental, also termed random, coincidences are events in which the LOR is incorrectly assigned due to two separate disintegrations occurring very closely

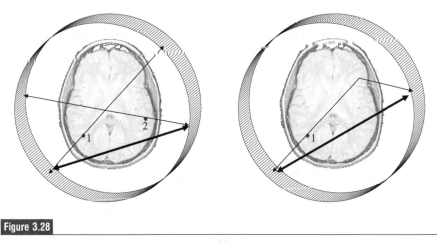

Figure 3.28

(left) An accidental coincidence recorded as an LOR between the first γ-rays hitting the detector ring from radioactive decays at positions 1 and 2 which occur very closely in time. (right) Incorrect LOR assigned from a scattered γ-ray.

in time. In one case, illustrated in Figure 3.28, the first γ-rays from each of the two events together form an incorrect LOR. A second possibility is that an incorrect LOR is formed due to one γ-ray being scattered, also shown in Figure 3.28. Accidental coincidences are uniformly distributed across the imaging field-of-view, and so can cause significant errors in areas which have very low activity. For clinical PET/CT head scanners accidental coincidences constitute ~20% of the attributed true coincidences, but for a body scanner the number can be closer to 50%.

The most common method of correcting for random coincidences uses additional parallel timing circuitry, in which a second coincidence timing window starts significantly later, typically 60 ns after an event is recorded. The standard circuit with a 6–12 ns resolving time is used to measure the total number of coincidences. The second measurement being delayed well beyond the coincidence resolving time means that only accidental coincidences are recorded. The accidental coincidences are then subtracted from the acquired data.

An alternative correction method is to measure the number of events recorded by each individual detector. If two detectors i and j are considered, then the rate at which accidental coincidences (C_{ij}^{acc}) are recorded is given by:

$$C_{ij}^{acc} = 2\tau R_i R_j, \tag{3.18}$$

where R_i and R_j are the single count rates in the individual detectors i and j, and 2τ is the coincidence resolving time. Therefore, the measured values of R_i and R_j for each detector pair i and j can be used to estimate the corresponding values of C_{ij}^{acc}, which are then subtracted from the acquired data. Multiple coincidences can also occur, in which more than two events are recorded during the coincidence resolving time. Estimates for the number of multiple coincidences (M_{ij}) between two detectors can be made using the expression:

$$M_{ij} \approx C_{ij}\tau R_{ij}N_{ij}, \tag{3.19}$$

where N_{ij} is the total number of detectors operating in coincidence with either of the two detectors i and j. Multiple event coincidences are simply discarded before image reconstruction.

3.18.3 Corrections for scattered coincidences

There are two major sources of scattered radiation that contaminate the PET signal, scatter within the body and scatter in the BGO detection crystal itself. BGO has a relatively poor intrinsic energy resolution, and the energy window is typically set to be between 450 and 650 keV for a clinical scan. Since a γ-ray that is scattered by 45° in the body only loses ~115 keV of its energy, scattered γ-rays represent a significant fraction of the detected γ-rays. In 2D PET, scattered γ-rays typically account for only ~10–15% of the detected signal, but in 3D mode up to 50% of the detected γ-rays can be scattered, this larger number due primarily to the elimination of the lead septa. The simplest method of correcting for scatter is to measure the signal intensity in areas that are outside the patient, and to fit these values to a Gaussian shape to estimate the amount of scatter inside the patient. This function is then subtracted from the raw data to give the corrected image. This approach works reasonably for relatively homogenous organs such as the brain, but cannot be used in the abdomen, for example. A second method is to use multiple energy window methods, as used in SPECT. The dual-energy window approach typically has the lower window set between 190 and 350 keV, with the upper window at 350–650 keV. An alternative method is termed the estimation of trues method (ETM) which also uses two windows, but in this case the lower window is 450–650 keV, which partially overlaps the upper window between 550 and 650 keV. The ETM makes the assumption that all of the events in the upper window arise from γ-rays that have not been scattered. These data are then scaled appropriately to equal the number of events recorded in the lower window, and these scaled data are then subtracted from the photopeak energy window. Finally, the most sophisticated but also most computationally intensive and time-consuming method is an iterative reconstruction based upon simulating the actual scatter using the CT-derived attenuation maps. The first estimate is simply formed from the data with no scatter correction: subsequent steps follow the type of iterative data flow already shown in Figure 3.16.

3.18.4 Corrections for dead time

As already outlined in Section 3.6.4, there is a maximum count rate that a system can record due to finite component response and recovery times. The fractional dead time of the PET system is defined as the ratio of the measured count rate to the theoretical count rate if the dead time were zero. The three major sources of deadtime in PET scanners are the time taken to integrate the charge from the PMTs after a scintillation event, the processing of a coincidence event, and the presence of multiple coincidences in which the data are discarded. Corrections are performed based mainly upon a careful characterization of the dead-time associated with each component of the PET system, and the number of multiple coincidences estimated using Equation (3.19).

3.19 Image characteristics

Signal-to-noise

Radiotracer dose, targeting efficiency, image acquisition time, γ-ray attenuation in the patient, system sensitivity and image post-processing play similar roles in determining the SNR in PET as they do in SPECT scans. As outlined earlier, the intrinsic sensitivity of PET is significantly greater than SPECT due to the lack of collimation requirements and the lower γ-ray attenuation in tissue of 511 keV γ-rays. In terms of the total number of γ-rays emitted by a particular radiotracer, approximately 0.01–0.03% are detected by a SPECT gamma camera, 0.2–0.5% in PET/CT using 2D acquisition-mode, and 2–10% in 3-D PET/CT. Due to the significant difference in sensitivity between 2D and 3D, many commercial PET/CT scanners now offer only 3D acquisition.

Contrast-to-noise

In addition to those factors affecting SNR, the CNR is mainly influenced by the correction for in Compton-scattered γ-rays, and the non-specific uptake of radiotracer in healthy tissue surrounding the pathology being studied, for example the uptake of FDG in brain, described further in Section 3.21.2.

Spatial resolution

In contrast to SPECT, in which the spatial resolution is significantly worse the deeper within the body that the radiotracer is located, the in-plane spatial resolution in PET is much more constant throughout the patient. This is because the inherent 'double detection' of two γ-rays in PET reduces the depth dependence of the PSF. Other factors which influence the spatial resolution of the PET image include:

(i) The effective positron range in tissue before it annihilates with an electron: this distance is longer the higher the energy of the emitted positron and the less dense the tissue through which it has to travel. Typical values of the maximum positron energy and corresponding FWHM distances travelled are: ^{18}F (640 keV, 0.2 mm), ^{11}C (960 keV, 0.4 mm), ^{13}N (1.2 MeV, 0.6 mm), ^{15}O (1.7 MeV, 1 mm), and ^{82}Rb (3.15 MeV, 2.6 mm),

(ii) The non-colinearity of the two γ-rays, i.e. the small random deviation from 180° of the angle of their relative trajectories. There is a distribution in angles about a mean of 180°, with a FHWM of approximately 0.5°. Therefore, the larger the diameter of the PET detector ring, the greater the effect this has on the spatial resolution, and

(iii) The dimensions of the detector crystals, with an approximate spatial resolution given by half the detector diameter. Since multiple Compton scattering interactions are required to 'stop' the γ-rays in the crystal there is also an uncertainty in the exact location at which the γ-ray first strikes the detector: this uncertainty increases with the thickness of the crystal, as seen previously.

The overall spatial resolution of the system is the combination of all three components:

$$R_{sys} \approx \sqrt{R_{detector}^2 + R_{range}^2 + R_{180^0}^2},\qquad(3.20)$$

with typical FWHM values of R_{sys} of 3–4 mm for a small ring system for brain studies, and 5–6 mm for a larger whole-body system.

3.20 Time-of-flight PET

The most recent development in commercial PET/CT scanners is that of time-of-flight (TOF) PET [10]. The concept of TOF PET, shown in Figure 3.29, is to constrain the estimated position of an annihilation to a subsection of the conventional LOR between two detectors by measuring the exact times at which the two γ-rays strike the detectors. Ideally, one would be able to constrain the position to a point, in which case spatial resolution would increase significantly. However, in order to do this, the timing accuracy of every scintillation event would have to be much less than 1 ns, which is not possible. Suppose that one has a timing resolution of Δt, then the position resolution, Δx, along a line between two detectors is given by:

$$\Delta x = \frac{c\Delta t}{2},\qquad(3.21)$$

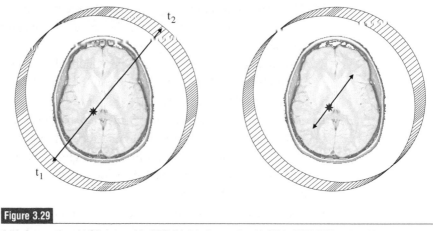

(left) Conventional LOR formed in PET. (right) Constrained LOR in TOF-PET defined by the time difference t_2-t_1 corresponding to the delay between the two γ-rays striking the particular detectors.

where c is the speed of light.

Commercial scanners are now available which offer TOF PET/CT as well as regular PET/CT. The scintillator used for the first commercial TOF PET systems is lutetium orthosilicate (LSO). Compared to BGO, LSO produces roughly three times the number of photons per MeV of energy absorbed, with only a slightly poorer energy resolution. Most importantly, the coincidence time (theoretically 450 ps, slightly greater in an actual PET system) is much shorter for LSO than for BGO (3 ns). A timing resolution of 500 ps corresponds to a spatial resolution of ~7.5 cm. Therefore, it would appear that TOF PET offers no advantages over conventional PET since the latter already has a spatial resolution of the order of several millimetres. However, being able to constrain the length of the LOR from its value in conventional PET to 7.5 cm reduces the statistical noise inherent in the measurement. Since the noise variance is proportional to the length of the LOR, the reduction in noise variance, the so-called multiplicative reduction factor (f), is given by:

$$f = \frac{D}{\Delta x} = \frac{2D}{c\Delta t}, \tag{3.22}$$

where D is the size of the patient. Since for both brain and whole-body imaging the value of D is much greater than 7.5 cm, the noise in TOF PET is reduced compared to conventional PET and the SNR is significantly enhanced. In a commercial scanner the crystal size of LSO is typically 4 $\times$ 4 mm, with a thickness of just over 2 cm. TOF PET/CT scanners incorporate either a 16- or 64-slice CT capability.

3.21   Clinical applications of PET/CT

PET/CT scans currently represent ~5–10% of all nuclear medicine scans, and are rapidly increasing in percentage each year. The majority (~90%) of PET/CT diagnoses are oncology scans using ^{18}FDG [11]. In the USA the Centers for Medicare Services have approved FDG PET/CT for reimbursement for, amongst others, lung, colorectal, oesophageal and head-and-neck cancers, as well as melanoma and lymphoma. Diagnoses of breast, thyroid and cervical cancer are also very promising areas which may be approved for medical reimbursement in the near future. PET/CT can also be used to follow the efficacy of cancer therapies. In addition, neurological conditions including seizure disorders and neurodegenerative diseases such as Alzheimer's and dementia can be assessed and monitored using PET/CT.

3.21.1   Whole-body PET/CT scanning

Malignant cells, in general, have higher rates of aerobic glucose metabolism than healthy cells. Therefore, in PET scans using FDG, tumours show up as areas of increased signal intensity provided that there is sufficient blood supply to deliver the radiotracer. When cancer, and in particular metastatic cancer in which the lesions have spread from their primary focus to secondary areas, is suspected a whole-body PET scan is performed. Patients either fast overnight for scans acquired in the morning, or for at least four hours before afternoon scans, since glucose competes with ^{18}FDG in terms of cellular uptake. A serum glucose level of ~150 mg/dl is the target value before injection. The patient is injected intravenously with ~10 mCi of FDG and scanned 30–60 minutes after this to allow most of the radiotracer to clear from the bloodstream and to accumulate in the tumour. A typical whole-body PET scan over a body length of 190 cm takes approximately 30 minutes, with the patient bed being moved a number of times within the scanner to cover the entire body. The most modern TOF PET/CT scanners can shorten the scanning time considerably. Figure 3.30 shows PET, CT and fused images from a whole-body scan.

3.21.2   PET/CT applications in the brain

Although FDG PET/CT can be used to diagnose brain tumours, the technique faces the challenge that there is a high background signal in the brain due to the natural metabolism of glucose in healthy brain tissue. Since the CNR is not high, the role

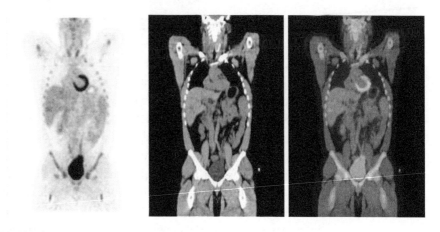

Figure 3.30

(left) Whole-body ^{18}FDG PET scan. (centre) Corresponding CT scan. (right) Fused PET/CT scan.

of the CT component of the hybrid scanner in defining the exact outline of the tumour is critical. The PET signal can then be used to grade the tumour by comparing the activitity within the tumour with that of surrounding white and grey brain matter. Low grade tumours typically have activity below that of white matter, whereas high grade tumours have levels equal to or even greater than those in grey matter. Figure 3.31 shows combined PET/CT images of the brain.

FDG PET is also used to characterize different types of neurodegenerative dementia such as Alzheimer's disease (AD) which is characterized by low

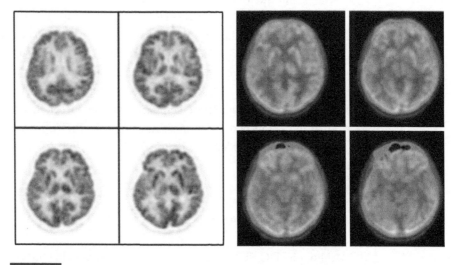

Figure 3.31

(left) ^{18}FDG PET scans of the brain. (right) Corresponding fused PET/CT images.

metabolism in the parietal and temporal lobes. Differentiation between AD and other dementias such as frontotemporal dementia can be made by characterizing the different extents of hypoactivity. Early evaluation of AD can also be performed with alternative targeted compounds. These include the so-called Pittsburgh Compound B (Pitt-B), which binds to amyloid proteins associated with amyloid plaque depositions in the brain. Areas of high signal intensity are found in the cortices where these plaques accumulate.

3.21.3 Cardiac PET/CT studies

Although SPECT is currently the most important diagnostic technique for myocardial viability and perfusion assessment, PET/CT is increasingly being used wherever it is available, primarily due to its higher spatial resolution (approximately 8 mm for PET versus 15 mm for SPECT) and the fact that one can perform cardiac-gated analysis of wall motion and ejection fraction. Myocardial perfusion PET/CT scans use either $^{13}NH_3$ or $^{82}RbCl_2$, with a similar stress test protocol to that performed for SPECT. Complementary PET viability studies are performed with ^{18}FDG which is preferentially taken up in myocardial cells which have poor perfusion but are metabolically active. In healthy myocardium long-chain fatty acids are the principal energy source, whereas in ischemic tissue glucose plays a major role in residual oxidative metabolism and the oxidation of long-chain fatty acids is reduced substantially. One example of the clinical application of cardiac PET is the assessment of whether a heart transplant or bypass surgery should be carried out on a particular patient. A measured absence of both blood flow and metabolism in parts of the heart show that the tissue has died, and so a heart transplant may be necessary. If blood flow is absent in an area, but the tissue maintains even a reduced metabolic state, then the tissue is still alive and bypass surgery would be more appropriate.

Exercises

Radioactivity
3.1 (a) In a sample of 20 000 atoms, if 400 decay in 8 seconds what is the radioactivity, measured in mCi, of the sample?

   (b) In order to produce a level of radioactivity of 1 mCi, how many nuclei of ^{99m}Tc ($\lambda = 3.22 \times 10^{-5}\,s^{-1}$) must be present? What mass of the radiotracer does this correspond to? (Avogadro's number is 6.02×10^{23}).

   (c) A radioactive sample of ^{99m}Tc contains 10 mCi activity at 9 am. What is the radioactivity of the sample at 12 pm on the same day?

3.2 In a nuclear medicine scan using ^{99m}Tc, the image SNR for a 30 minute scan was 25:1 for an injected radioactive dose of 1 mCi. Imaging began immediately after injection.

(a) If the injected dose were tripled to 3 mCi, what would be the image SNR for a 30 minute scan?

(b) If the scan time were doubled to 60 minutes with an initial dose of 1 mCi, what would be the image SNR?

3.3 A dose of 1 mCi of ^{99m}Tc is administered to a patient. Calculate the total dose to the patient if the biological half-life of the radiotracer in the body is:

(a) 2 years,

(b) 6 hours,

(c) 2 minutes.

The technetium generator.

3.4 In the technetium generator, show mathematically that if $\lambda_2 \gg \lambda_1$, the radioactivities of the parent and daughter nuclei become equal in value at long times.

3.5 Using the equations derived in the analysis of the technetium generator, plot graphs of the activity of parent and daughter nuclei for the following cases:

(a) $\tau_{1/2}$ (parent) = 600 hours, $\tau_{1/2}$ (daughter) = 6 hours,

(b) $\tau_{1/2}$ (parent) = 6.1 hours, $\tau_{1/2}$ (daughter) = 6 hours,

(c) $\tau_{1/2}$ (parent) = 0.6 hours, $\tau_{1/2}$ (daughter) = 6 hours.

3.6 Calculate the exact time at which the first three 'milkings' of the technetium cow should be performed.

3.7 Do the tops of the curves in Figure 3.4 lie at the same values that would have been obtained if the technetium cow were not milked at all?

3.8 Rather than waiting 24 hours, only 6 hours are left between milkings. Plot the graph of radioactivity over the first two days.

The gamma camera.

3.9 Calculate the magnification factor for the pinhole collimator shown in Figure 3.32(a). What implications does this have for image distortions?

3.10 If the acceptance window for a planar nuclear medicine scan is set to 15%, what is the maximum angle that a γ-ray could be Compton scattered and still be accepted if it strikes the scintillation crystal?

3.11 What is the energy of a γ-ray which has been Compton scattered at an angle of 30° in the body?

3.12 (i) The thickness of the lead septa is chosen to ensure that only 5% of the γ-rays penetrate from one collimator hole to the adjacent one. Using Figure 3.32(b) show that the thickness is given by $[6d/\mu]/[L-3/\mu]$.

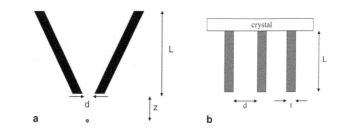

Figure 3.32

See Exercise 3.9.

PMT	R_{X+} (Ω)	R_{X-} (Ω)	R_{Y+} (Ω)	R_{Y-} (Ω)
8	infinite	14.3	28.6	28.6
9	57.1	19.0	28.6	28.6
10	28.6	28.6	28.6	28.6
11	19.0	57.1	28.6	28.6
12	14.3	infinite	28.6	28.6

(ii) Calculate the septal thickness required for γ-rays of 140 keV for lead collimators with a hole diameter of 0.1 cm and a length of 2.5 cm. The attenuation coefficient for lead is 30 cm^{-1} at 140 keV.

3.13 Assuming that the body is circular with a diameter of 30 cm, calculate the spatial resolution (FWHM) for a parallel hole collimator, length 2.5 cm, for two sources of radioactivity, one very close to the detector ($z = 0$) and one at the other side of the body ($z \sim 30$).

3.14 Stating any assumptions that you make, show that for the parallel collimator there is an approximate relationship between collimator efficiency and spatial resolution given by:

$$g \propto R_{coll}^2.$$

3.15 For the converging collimator shown in Figure 3.33 describe qualitatively (without mathematical proof) (i) whether the efficiency increases or decreases as a function of z, and as a function of θ, and (ii) whether the resolution increases or decreases as a function of θ, and as a function of z.

3.16 Given the following resistor values for the Anger network, show that the output is linear in X.

Image characteristics

3.17 Three parameters which affect the image SNR in nuclear medicine are the thickness of the detector crystal, the length of the lead septa in the anti-scatter

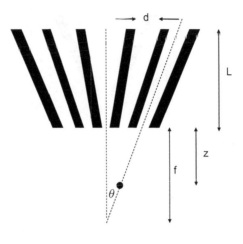

Figure 3.33

See Exercise 3.15.

grid, and the FWHM of the energy window centred around 140 keV. For each parameter, does an increase in the value of the particular parameter increase or decrease the image SNR? In each case, name one other image characteristic (e.g. CNR, spatial resolution) that is affected, and explain whether this image characteristic is improved or degraded.

3.18 Suppose that two radiotracers could be given to a patient. Radiotracer A is taken up in a tumour ten times higher than in the surrounding tissue, whereas B suppresses uptake by a factor of 10. Assume the tumour is 1 cm thickness and the surrounding tissue is 10 cm thickness. Ignoring attenuation effects, what is the CNR generated from each tumour. Assume that the uptake in normal tissue gives a rate of 10 counts per minute per cubic centimetre of tissue, and that the imaging time is 1 minute.

SPECT

3.19 Isosensitive imaging is a technique that acquires nuclear medicine scans from opposite sides of the patient, and then combines the signals to remove the depth dependence of the signal intensity. By considering the attenuation of γ-rays in the patient, show how this technique works, and what mathematical processing of the two scans is necessary.

3.20 For a 64 × 64 data matrix, how many total counts are necessary for a 10% pixel-by-pixel uniformity level in a SPECT image?

3.21 Answer true or false with a couple of sentences of explanation. If a uniform attenuation correction is applied to a SPECT scan, a tumour positioned close to bone appears to have a lower radioactivity than is actually the true situation.

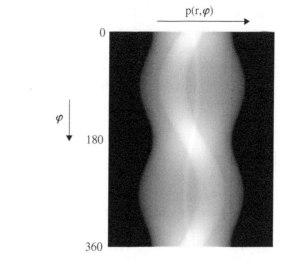

$p(r,\varphi)$

0

φ

180

360

Figure 3.34

See Exercise 3.22.

3.22 A SPECT scan is taken of a patient, and areas of radioactivity are found. The sinogram from the SPECT scan is shown in Figure 3.34. What are the shapes of the areas of radioactivity?

3.23 Calculate the maximum angle and corresponding energy of Compton scattered γ-rays accepted for energy resolutions of 5, 15 and 25%.

PET

3.24 Using the rest mass of the electron, show that the energies of the two γ-rays produced by the annihilation of an electron with a positron are 511 keV.

3.25 PET scans often show an artificially high level of radioactivity in the lungs. Suggest one mechanism by which this might occur.

3.26 For an ^{15}O PET scan, if an initial dose of 1 mCi is injected, calculate the total number of γ-rays that are produced over a scan time of 4 minutes, assuming that scanning starts immediately after injection, and that clearance from the body is negligible.

3.27 What timing resolution would be necessary to obtain a position resolution of 5 mm in TOF PET based only upon time-of-flight considerations?

3.28 If the brain is assumed to be a sphere with diameter 20 cm, and the largest dimension of the body to be 40 cm, what are the respective values of the timing resolution necessary to reduce the noise in TOF PET compared to conventional PET?

3.29 Suggest why a PET/CT scanner operating in 2D mode has a relatively uniform axial sensitivity profile, whereas in 3D mode the sensitivity is much higher at the centre of the scanner.

3.30 Suggest why a curvilinear region of low signal intensity is often seen on PET/CT scans of the thorax and abdomen, which parallels the dome of the diaphragm.

References

[1] Anger H. Scintillation camera. *Review of Scientific Instruments* 1958;**29**,27–33.

[2] O'Connor MK and Kemp BJ. Single-photon emission computed tomography/ Computed tomography: Basic instrumentation and innovations. *Seminars in Nuclear Medicine* 2006:**36**, 258–66.

[3] Seo Y, Mari C and Hasegawa BH. Technological development and advances in single-photon emission computed tomography/computed tomography. *Seminars in Nuclear Medicine* 2008:**38**, 177–198.

[4] Robertson JS, Marr RB, Rosenblum M, Radeka V and Yamamoto YL. Thirty-two-crystal positron transverse section detector. In: Freedmen GS, editor. *Tomographic imaging in nuclear medicine.* New York: Society of Nuclear Medicine; 1973: 142–53.

[5] Ter-Pogossian MM, Mullani NA, Hood J, Higgins CS and Curie M. A multi-slice postitron emission computed tomograph (PETT IV) yielding transverse and longitudinal images. *Radiology* 1978:**128**, 477–484.

[6] Rahmin A and Zaidi H. PET vs. SPECT: strengths, limitations and challenges. *Nuclear Medicine Communications* 2008:**29**, 193–207.

[7] Mittra E and Quon A. Positron emission tomography/computed tomography: the current technology and applications. *Radiological Clinics of North America* 2009:**47**, 147–60.

[8] Gallagher GM, Ansari A, Atkins H et al. Radiopharmaceuticals XXVII. 18F-labeled 2-deoxy-2-fluoro-D-glucose as a radiopharmaceutical for measuring regional myocardial glucose metabolism in vivo: tissue distribution and imaging studies in animals. *Journal of Nuclear Medicine* 1977: **18**, 990–6.

[9] van Eijk CWE. Radiation detector developments in medical applications: inorganic scintillators in positron emission tomography. *Radiation Protection Dosimetry* 2008:**129**, 13–21.

[10] Moses WM. Recent advances and future advances in time-of-flight PET. *Nuclear Instrument Methods Physics Research A* 2007:**580**, 919–24.

[11] Pan T and Mawlawi O. PET/CT in radiation oncology. *Medical Physics* 2008:**35**, 4955–66.

4 Ultrasound imaging

4.1 Introduction

Of all the standard clinical imaging techniques ultrasound is by far the least expensive and most portable (including handheld units smaller than a laptop computer), and can acquire continuous images at a real-time frame rate with few or no safety concerns. In addition to morphological and structural information, ultrasound can also measure blood flow in real-time, and produce detailed maps of blood velocity within a given vessel. Ultrasound finds very wide use in obstetrics and gynaecology, due to the lack of ionizing radiation or strong magnetic fields. The real-time nature of the imaging is also important in measuring parameters such as foetal heart function. Ultrasound is used in many cardiovascular applications, being able to detect mitral valve and septal insufficiencies. General imaging applications include liver cysts, aortic aneurysms, and obstructive atherosclerosis in the carotids. Ultrasound imaging is also used very often to guide the path and positioning of a needle in tissue biopsies.

Ultrasound is a mechanical wave, with a frequency for clinical use between 1 and 15 MHz. The speed of sound in tissue is ~1540 m/s, and so the range of wavelengths of ultrasound in tissue is between ~0.1 and 1.5 mm. The ultrasound waves are produced by a transducer, as shown in Figure 4.1, which typically has an array of up to 512 individual active sources. In the simplest image acquisition scheme, small subgroups of these elements are fired sequentially to produce parallel ultrasound beams. As the ultrasound passes through tissue, a small fraction of the energy is reflected from the boundaries between tissues which have slightly different acoustic and physical properties: the remaining energy of the beam is transmitted through the boundary. The reflected waves are detected by the transducer and the distance to each tissue boundary is calculated from the time between pulse transmission and signal reception: thus ultrasound imaging is very similar to techniques such as radar. As soon as the signal from the deepest tissue boundary has been detected from one beam, the next adjacent beam of ultrasound is emitted, and this process is repeated until the entire image has been acquired. Due to the relatively high speed of ultrasound through tissue, entire images can be

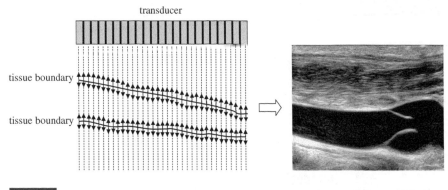

transducer

tissue boundary

tissue boundary

(left) Basic principle of ultrasound imaging. A transducer sends a series of pressure waves through the tissue. At boundaries between tissues, a small fraction of the energy is backscattered towards the transducer where it is detected. Using the speed of sound through tissue, the depth of the tissue boundary can be determined. Electronic steering of the beam across the sample builds up successive lines which form the image. (right) The intensity of each pixel in the image is proportional to the strength of the detected signal reflected from that point.

acquired in fractions of a second, allowing real-time imaging to be performed. Ultrasound imaging can also be used to measure blood flow via the Doppler effect, in which the frequency of the received signal is slightly different than that of the transmitted signal due to blood flow either towards or away from the transducer.

Advances in instrumentation have made extraordinary improvements in image quality possible over the past decade. As examples of such advances, transducers are now able to cover very large frequency bandwidths enabling harmonic imaging to be performed efficiently. Two-dimensional transducers allow three-dimensional ultrasound to be performed in real-time. The incorporation of digital electronics into receiver beam-forming, and new data acquisition techniques such as pulse inversion imaging have improved image quality significantly. In addition, the development of new ultrasound contrast agents based on microbubbles can increase the signal intensity from flowing blood by orders of magnitude.

4.2 Wave propagation and characteristic acoustic impedance

A simple model of tissue to illustrate the principles of ultrasound propagation is a three-dimensional lattice of small particles held together by elastic forces. The ultrasound transducer transmits a pressure wave into tissue with a broad band of frequencies centred at its specified operating frequency. Passage of energy through the tissue causes individual particles to oscillate about their mean positions. As

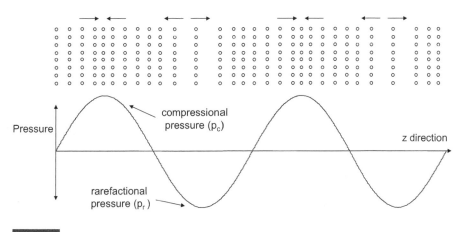

Figure 4.2

The effect of the passage of an ultrasound wave on the displacement of the molecules within tissue. The maximum positive pressure of the wave corresponds to the maximum compressional force, pushing the molecules together. The corresponding maximum negative pressure represents a rarefactional force.

with all types of wave propagation, the distances moved by the individual particles are very small compared to the overall distance travelled by the pressure wave. In ultrasound imaging the directions of particle vibration and wave propagation are the same, meaning that the ultrasound can be considered as a purely longitudinal wave, as shown in Figure 4.2.

For typical ultrasound frequencies (1–15 MHz) used in clinical diagnosis, the value of the particle displacement, W, is a few tenths of a nanometer. The speed (c) of the ultrasound wave through tissue is determined by the tissue density (ρ) and compressibility (κ) values:

$$c = \frac{1}{\sqrt{\kappa\rho}}. \tag{4.1}$$

Equation (4.1) shows that the more rigid the tissue and/or the less dense the tissue, the higher the ultrasound propagation velocity. Table 4.1 shows that the value of c in most soft tissues is approximately 1540 m/s. The values in bone and air (e.g. lungs) represent the two extremes due to highly disparate density and compressibility.

The particle velocity (u_z) along the direction of energy propagation (denoted as the z-direction here) is given by the time derivative of the particle displacement:

$$u_z = \frac{dW}{dt}. \tag{4.2}$$

Table 4.1: Acoustic properties of biological tissues

	$Z \times 10^5$ (g cm^{-2} s^{-1})	Speed of sound (m s^{-1})	Density (gm^{-3})	Compressibility $\times 10^{11}$ (cm g^{-1} s^2)
Air	0.00043	330	1.3	70 000
Blood	1.59	1570	1060	4.0
Bone	7.8	4000	1908	0.3
Fat	1.38	1450	925	5.0
Brain	1.58	1540	1025	4.2
Muscle	1.7	1590	1075	3.7
Liver	1.65	1570	1050	3.9
Kidney	1.62	1560	1040	4.0

The value of u_z is approximately 0.01 m s^{-1}, and is much lower than the value of c. The pressure (p), measured in pascals (Pa), of the ultrasound wave at a particular point in the z-direction is given by:

$$p = \rho c u_z. \tag{4.3}$$

Positive pressure corresponds to compressional forces and negative pressure to rarefactional forces, as shown in Figure 4.2. A particularly important parameter in ultrasound imaging is the characteristic acoustic impedance (Z) of tissue, which is defined as the ratio of the pressure to the particle velocity:

$$Z = \frac{p}{u_z}. \tag{4.4}$$

This equation can be considered as a direct analogue to Ohm's law in an electrical circuit. A voltage driving force produces a current, with the ratio between the two quantities being determined by the circuit impedance. Therefore, the complementary physical constants are voltage/pressure, current/particle velocity, and impedance/characteristic impedance. The value of Z is determined by the physical properties of the tissue:

$$Z = \rho c = \rho \frac{1}{\sqrt{\rho \kappa}} = \sqrt{\frac{\rho}{\kappa}}. \tag{4.5}$$

Table 4.1 also lists values of Z for tissues relevant to clinical ultrasound imaging. The values of Z for many soft tissues are very similar to one another, with again the two major differences being for lung tissue (air) and bone which have much lower and higher values, respectively. The next section explains how the Z values affect the propagation of ultrasound energy through the body.

Example 4.1   Given the values of c = 1540 m s^{-1} and ρ = 1.05 g cm^{-3} for brain tissue, calculate the values of the characteristic acoustic impedance and compressibility.

Solution   The characteristic impedance of brain tissue is given by:

$$Z = \rho c = 1.05(\text{g cm}^{-3}) \times 154000(\text{cm s}^{-1}) = 1.58 \times 10^5 \text{g cm}^{-2}\text{s}^{-1}.$$

From Equation (4.5), $Z^2 = \rho/\kappa$ and so:

$$\kappa = \rho/Z^2 = 1.05(\text{g cm}^{-3})/(1.58 \times 10^5)^2\text{g}^2 \text{cm}^{-4}\text{s}^{-2}$$
$$= 4.2 \times 10^{-11} \text{ cm g}^{-1}\text{s}^2.$$

Using the SI definition of 1 Pascal (Pa) as 1 kg m^{-1} s^{-2}, which is equivalent to 10 g cm^{-1} s^{-2}, the units of compressibility are the same as inverse pressure.

4.3   Wave reflection, refraction and scattering in tissue

As the ultrasound beam passes through tissue it encounters different tissues with different acoustic properties, as shown in Table 4.1. Whenever either a boundary between two tissues, or small structures within a homogeneous tissue, are encountered the differences in acoustic properties result in a fraction of the energy of the ultrasound beam being backscattered towards the transducer, where it forms the detected signal.

4.3.1   Reflection, transmission and refraction at tissue boundaries

When an ultrasound wave encounters a boundary between two tissues with different values of Z, a certain fraction of the wave energy is backscattered (or reflected) towards the transducer, with the remainder being transmitted through the boundary deeper into the body. In the first case considered here, the boundary is shown in Figure 4.3 as being flat, implying that its dimensions are much greater than the ultrasound wavelength, for example ≫ 1 mm for a 1.5 MHz central frequency. In the general situation shown in Figure 4.3, the incident ultrasound wave strikes the boundary at an angle θ_i.

The following equations relate the angles of incidence (θ_i) and reflection (θ_r), angles of incidence (θ_i) and transmission (θ_t), reflected (p_r) and transmitted (p_t) pressures, and reflected (I_r) and transmitted (I_t) intensities:

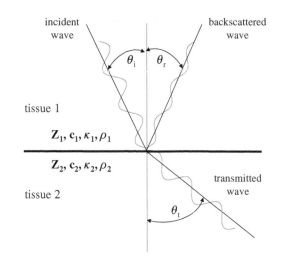

Showing the behaviour of an ultrasound beam when it strikes the boundary between two tissues with different acoustic properties. A certain fraction of the wave is backscattered/reflected back towards the transducer, with the remaining fraction being transmitted through the boundary deeper into tissue.

$$\theta_i = \theta_r, \tag{4.6}$$

$$\frac{\sin\theta_i}{\sin\theta_t} = \frac{c_1}{c_2}, \tag{4.7}$$

$$R_p = \frac{p_r}{p_i} = \frac{Z_2 \cos\theta_i - Z_1 \cos\theta_t}{Z_2\cos\theta_i + Z_1\cos\theta_t}, \tag{4.8}$$

$$T_p = \frac{p_t}{p_i} = \frac{2Z_2 \cos\theta_i}{Z_2 \cos\theta_i + Z_1 \cos\theta_t}, \tag{4.9}$$

$$R_I = \frac{I_r}{I_i} = \frac{(Z_2 \cos\theta_i - Z_1 \cos\theta_t)^2}{(Z_2 \cos\theta_i + Z_1 \cos\theta_t)^2}, \tag{4.10}$$

$$T_I = \frac{I_t}{I_i} = \frac{4Z_2 Z_1 \cos^2\theta_i}{(Z_2 \cos\theta_i + Z_1 \cos\theta_t)^2}. \tag{4.11}$$

The values of the reflection and transmission pressure coefficents are related by:

$$T_p = R_p + 1, \tag{4.12}$$

with the corresponding values of intensity reflection coefficients given by:

$$T_I = 1 - |R_I|^2. \tag{4.13}$$

Equation (4.7) shows that the ~~values of θ_i and θ_t are very similar~~, except in the case of the wave encountering a tissue/bone or tissue/air interface in which case a ~~significant deviation in the trajectory of the beam will occur~~. This produces a geometric artifact in the images in which tissues appear slightly displaced compared to their actual physical location within the body.

The strongest reflected signal is received if the angle between the incident wave and the boundary is 90°. In this case, Equations (4.8–4.11) reduce to:

$$R_p = \frac{p_r}{p_i} = \frac{Z_2 - Z_1}{Z_2 + Z_1}, \tag{4.14}$$

$$T_p = \frac{p_t}{p_i} = \frac{2Z_2}{Z_2 + Z_1}, \tag{4.15}$$

$$R_I = \frac{I_r}{I_i} = R_p^2 = \frac{(Z_2 - Z_1)^2}{(Z_2 + Z_1)^2}, \tag{4.16}$$

$$T_I = \frac{I_t}{I_i} = \frac{4Z_1 Z_2}{(Z_1 + Z_2)^2}. \tag{4.17}$$

The ~~backscattered signal detected by the~~ transducer is maximized if the value of either ~~Z_1 or Z_2 is zero~~. However, in this case the ~~ultrasound beam~~ will not reach structures that ~~lie deeper~~ in the body. Such a case occurs, for example, in ~~GI tract imaging if the ultrasound beam encounters pockets of air~~. A very strong signal is received from the front of the air pocket, but there is no information of clinical relevance from any structures behind the air pocket. At the other extreme, if Z_1 and Z_2 are equal in value, then there is no backscattered signal at all and the tissue boundary is essentially undetectable. Using values of Z in Table 4.1 and the reflection and transmission equations, it can be seen that, at boundaries between soft tissues, the intensity of the reflected wave is typically less than 0.1% of that of the incident wave.

Example 4.2   Calculate the angle of refraction for ultrasound with an incident angle of 20° striking the interface between lipid and muscle.

Solution   Using Equation (4.7), the angle can be calculated from:

$$\frac{\sin 20}{\sin \theta_t} = \frac{1450}{1590},$$

which gives a value of θ_t of 22°.

It is instructive to consider the values of R_p, T_p, R_I and T_I for three cases:

(i) $Z_1 \gg Z_2$, e.g. the ultrasound beam travels from tissue into air. The value of T_p is 0, T_i is 0, R_I is 1 and R_p is -1. The negative sign for R_p signifies that the backscattered pressure wave undergoes a 180° phase shift at the point at which it encounters the boundary.

(ii) $Z_1 \sim Z_2$, e.g. the ultrasound beam encounters a liver/kidney interface. In this case $T_r \sim 1$, $R_p < 1$, $T_I \sim 1$, $R_I \ll 1$. The backscattered signal is small in amplitude, but most of the ultrasound beam is transmitted through the boundary and so reaches tissues deeper in the body.

(iii) $Z_1 \ll Z_2$, e.g. the ultrasound beam travels from tissue into bone. In this case $T_I = 0$, $R_I = 1$, $T_r = 1$ and $R_p = 2$! The somewhat surprising value of $R_p = 2$ means that the pressure at a single point at the boundary is actually twice that of the incident wave. As in case (i), almost all of the energy is reflected back towards the transducer, except that there is no phase shift.

4.3.2 Scattering by small structures

In contrast to reflection and refraction at a tissue boundary which is much larger than the ultrasound wavelength, if the ultrasound beam strikes structures which are approximately the same size as, or smaller than, the ultrasound wavelength then the wave is scattered in all directions. The angular dependence (predominantly forwards, backwards or random) and magnitude of the scattered beam depend upon the shape, size and physical and acoustic properties (Z, κ, ρ) of the structure. If the size of the scattering body is small compared to the wavelength, then scattering is relatively uniform in direction, with slightly more energy being scattered back towards the transducer than away from it. In this size regime, referred to as Rayleigh scattering and shown in Figure 4.4, the amount of scattered energy increases as the fourth power of frequency. An example is the scattering of ultrasound by red blood cells, which have a diameter of the order of 5–10 μm. Since the red blood cells are very close to one another, as shown in Figure 4.4 (b), scattering patterns from individual red blood cells add constructively. This phenomenon is the basis of Doppler ultrasound, covered in Section 4.10, which is an extremely important method of measuring blood flow in many clinical diagnostic protocols. In contrast, if the scattering structures are relatively far apart, as shown in Figure 4.4 (c), then the resulting pattern is a complicated combination of constructive and destructive interference, known as speckle. Although speckle does have some information content, in general it is

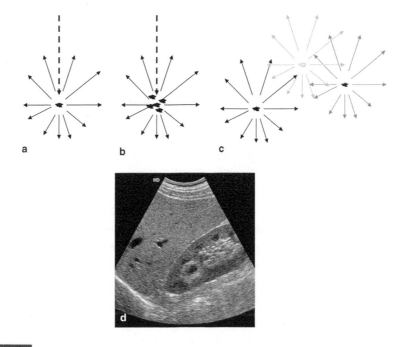

Figure 4.4

(a) Rayleigh scattering of an ultrasound beam by a structure which is physically small compared to the wavelength of the ultrasound beam. (b) Scattering from several structures which are close together produces scattered waves which add constructively. (c) Scattering structures which are relatively far from one another produce scattering patterns which add constructively at certain locations and destructively at others, thus producing areas of high and low image intensity, as illustrated in the image in (d).

considered to be an undesirable 'noise' component in ultrasound imaging, and techniques such as compound imaging (covered in Section 4.8.4) have been designed to reduce its contribution. Figure 4.4 shows an ultrasound image which shows examples of both distinct tissue boundaries and speckle within tissue.

4.4 Absorption and total attenuation of ultrasound energy in tissue

As an ultrasound beam passes through the body, its energy is attenuated by a number of mechanisms including reflection and scatter as covered in the previous section, and absorption covered next. The net effect is that signals received from tissue boundaries deep in the body are much weaker than those from boundaries which lie close to the surface.

4.4.1 Relaxation and classical absorption

In addition to backscattering from boundaries and small structures, the intensity of the ultrasound beam is reduced by absorption, which converts the energy of the beam into heat. There are two mechanisms by which such energy absorption takes place in biological tissue. The more important is termed 'relaxation absorption'.

Different tissues have different elastic properties, which can be quantitatively described by a relaxation time (τ), which characterizes the time that structures within the tissue require to return to their equilibrium position after having been displaced (either compressed or rarefacted) by the ultrasound wave. As an example, shown in Figure 4.2, consider that the positive component of the pressure wave moves the particles to the right, whereas the negative component of the pressure wave moves them in the opposite direction. After passage of the maximum positive component of the pressure wave, the elastic forces within the tissue pull the particles back towards the left. If the relaxation time is such that this motion coincides with the passage of the maximum negative pressure (which also moves the particles to the left), then these two forces act constructively and relatively little energy is extracted from the ultrasound beam. In contrast, if the relaxation time is such that the restoring elastic forces are moving the particle to the left at the same time as the passage of the next positive pressure maximum, which tries to move the particle to the right, then a much larger amount of energy is lost from the beam. A useful analogy is that of pushing a swing: the minimum energy required occurs when one pushes in the same direction that the swing is moving at the lowest point of its trajectory (when the velocity is highest), and the maximum energy required corresponds to the same point in its trajectory but when it is travelling in the opposite direction.

The relaxation process is characterized by a relaxation absorption coefficient, β_r, which is given by:

$$\beta_r = \frac{B_0 f^2}{1 + \left(f / f_r \right)^2}.$$

(4.18)

A graph of β_r as a function of frequency is shown in Figure 4.5, with a maximum value at f_r, the relaxation frequency, which is equal to $1/\tau$. Higher values of β_r correspond to more energy being absorbed in the body. In reality, tissue contains a broad range of values of τ and f_R, and the overall absorption coefficient is proportional to the sum of all the individual contributions:

$$\beta_{r,\text{tissue}} \propto \sum_n \frac{f^2}{1 + \left(f / f_{r,n} \right)^2}.$$

(4.19)

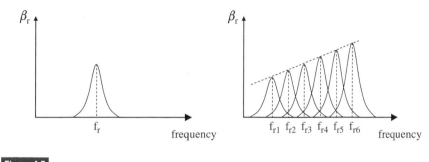

Figure 4.5

Plots of the relaxation absorption coefficient, β_r, for a completely homogeneous tissue (left) and for a realistic tissue (right) in which there are many relaxation frequencies. The overall absorption coefficient increases linearly with frequency.

Measured values of absorption in many tissues have shown that there is an almost linear relationship between the total absorption coefficient and ultrasound operating frequency, as shown in Figure 4.5.

There is a second, less important, mechanism for energy absorption called classical absorption. This effect is caused by friction between particles as they are displaced by the passage of the ultrasound wave. This loss is characterized by an absorption coefficient, β_{class}, which is proportional to the square of the operating frequency. The overall absorption coefficient is a combination of relaxation and classical absorption, but in biological tissues at clinical frequencies, the former mechanism is dominant.

4.4.2 Attenuation coefficients

Attenuation of the ultrasound beam as it propagates through tissue is the sum of absorption and scattering from small structures. Attenuation is characterized by an exponential decrease in both the pressure and intensity of the ultrasound beam as a function of its propagation distance, z, through tissue:

$$
\begin{aligned}
I(z) &= I(z = 0)e^{-\mu z} \\
p(z) &= p(z = 0)e^{-\alpha z},
\end{aligned}
\tag{4.20}
$$

where μ is the intensity attenuation coefficient and α is the pressure attenuation coefficient, both measured in units of cm^{-1}. The value of μ is equal to twice that of α. The value of μ is often stated in units of decibels (dB) per cm, where the conversion factor between the two units is given by:

$$\mu(\text{dB cm}^{-1}) = 4.343\mu(\text{cm}^{-1}). \qquad (4.21)$$

A useful rule-of-thumb is that each 3 dB reduction corresponds to a reduction in intensity by a factor of 2. So a 6 dB reduction corresponds to a factor of 4, a 9 dB reduction to a factor of 8 and so on.

The frequency dependence of μ for soft tissue is 1 dB cm^{-1} MHz^{-1}, i.e. at 2 MHz the attenuation coefficient is 2 dB cm^{-1}. For fat the attenuation coefficient is given approximately by $0.7f^{1.5}$ dB. The values of the attenuation coefficient for air and bone are much higher, 45 dB cm^{-1}MHz^{-1} and 8.7 dB cm^{-1} MHz^{-1}, respectively.

Example 4.3   The intensity of a 3 MHz ultrasound beam entering tissue is 10 mW/cm^2. Calculate the intensity at a depth of 4 cm.

Solution   The attenuation coefficient is 1 dB cm^{-1} MHz^{-1}, and so has a value of 3 dB cm^{-1} at 3 MHz. At a depth of 4 cm, the attenuation is 12 dB, which corresponds to a factor of 16. So the intensity of the beam is 0.625 mW/cm^2.

4.5   Instrumentation

A block-diagram of the basic instrumentation used for ultrasound imaging is shown in Figure 4.6. The input signal to the transducer comes from a frequency generator. The frequency generator is gated on for short time durations and then gated off, thus producing short periodic voltage pulses. These pulsed voltage signals are amplified and fed via a transmit/receive switch to the transducer. Since the transducer both transmits high power pulses and also receives very low intensity signals, the transmit and receive circuits must be very well isolated from each other; this is the purpose of the transmit/receive switch. The amplified voltage is converted by the transducer into a mechanical pressure wave which is transmitted into the body. Reflection and scattering from boundaries and structures within tissue occur, as described previously. The backscattered pressure waves reach the transducer at different times dictated by the depth in tissue from which they originate, and are converted into voltages by the transducer. These voltages have relatively small values, and so pass through a very low-noise preamplifier before being digitized. Time-gain compensation (Section 4.7.5) is used to reduce the dynamic range of the signals, and after appropriate further amplification and signal processing, the images are displayed in real time on the computer monitor.

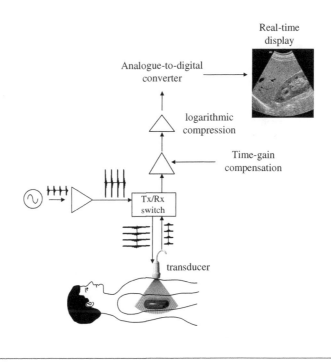

Figure 4.6

The major elements of a basic ultrasound imaging system.

Additional circuitry in both the transmit and receive channels is required when using phased array transducers, and this is covered in Sections 4.7.3 and 4.7.4.

4.6 Single element ultrasound transducers

Although the vast majority of transducers consist of a large array of small elements, it is useful to consider first the properties of a single element transducer, shown schematically in Figure 4.7. Shaped piezoelectric material is the active element of all ultrasound transducers, and is formed from a composite of lead zirconate titanate (PZT). Fine powders of the three metal oxides are mixed and then heated to high temperatures ($> 120\,°C$) and placed in a strong electric field, with a value of tens of kV per cm. This field aligns the dipoles within the material, and confers the property of being piezoelectric, i.e. able to convert an oscillating voltage to changes in physical dimension, and vice versa. Thin rods of PZT are embedded in a resin, and the material is then formed into the required shape and size. In the case of a single element transducer, the element is usually disk-shaped or formed into a spherical or cylindrical shell. The two faces of the element are coated with a thin layer of silver and connected via bonding wires to a coaxial cable leading to the

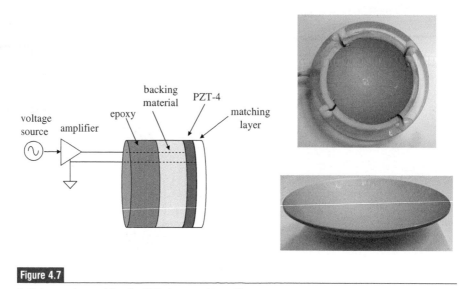

Figure 4.7

(left) A transducer with a flat PZT element. (right) Flat and hemispherical PZT elements.

transmit-receive switch. Examples of flat and curved PZT elements are shown in Figure 4.7.

When an oscillating voltage is applied to one face of the piezoelectric element, its thickness oscillates at the same frequency as the applied voltage, with the change in thickness being proportional to the magnitude and polarity of this voltage up to the maximum displacement of the transducer (a higher driving voltage can cause damage). Placing the element in physical contact with a patient's skin transfers the mechanical motion of the piezoelectric element into a pressure wave which is transmitted into the body.

The element has a natural resonant frequency (f_0) corresponding to its thickness (t) being one-half of the wavelength of ultrasound in the crystal

$$t = \frac{\lambda_{crystal}}{2} = \frac{c_{crystal}}{2f_0} \Rightarrow f_0 = \frac{c_{crystal}}{2t}. \tag{4.22}$$

The value of $c_{crystal}$ in a PZT crystal is approximately 4000 m s^{-1}, and so the thickness of a crystal for operation at 3 MHz is ~1.3 mm.

As shown in Equation (4.10), the larger the difference in the characteristic acoustic impedance of two materials, the greater the intensity of the reflected wave from the boundary between the two. A PZT-based transducer has a Z value of ~30 × 10^5 g cm^{-2} s^{-1}, compared to the value of skin/tissue of ~1.7 × 10^5 g cm^{-2} s^{-1}. Therefore, without some modifications, there would be a large amount of energy reflected from the patient's skin, and the efficiency of coupling the mechanical wave into the body would be very low. To improve this efficiency, a 'matching layer' is added to the external face of the crystal to provide acoustic coupling between the crystal and the patient. Intuitively, one can imagine that the value of Z of this matching layer ($Z_{matching\ layer}$) should be intermediate between that of the transducer element (Z_{PZT}) and the skin (Z_{skin}). In fact the value is given by the geometric mean of the two Z-values (see Exercise 4.7):

$$Z_{matching\ layer} = \sqrt{Z_{PZT}Z_{skin}}. \tag{4.23}$$

The thickness of this matching layer should be one-quarter of the ultrasound wavelength, to maximize energy transmission through the layer in both directions (see Exercise 4.10). Although the matching layer improves the transmission efficiency (and also reception) it does not provide 100% efficiency, and so many manufacturers use multiple matching layers to increase the efficiency further.

As shown in Figure 4.7, the PZT element is mechanically coupled to a damping layer consisting of a backing material and epoxy. In ultrasound imaging a number of short pulses of ultrasound energy are sent into the body. As covered later in Section 4.6.3, the axial spatial resolution (i.e. along the direction of the ultrasound beam) is proportional to the total length of the ultrasound pulse, and so a short pulse is required for good spatial resolution. The output of the frequency generator is gated on for a short period of time, typically comprising two to three cycles of the particular frequency for each pulse. If no mechanical damping is used, then the PZT element will 'ring' after the end of the voltage pulse, thus producing a pulse of ultrasound energy which is much longer than the applied voltage pulse, as shown in Figure 4.8, resulting in poor axial resolution. A familiar analogy would be the long sound produced from a single strike of a bell. Adding some mechanical damping reduces the length of the sound. A similar effect is achieved in an ultrasound transducer. Efficient damping is also important in terms of achieving a large frequency bandwidth, as covered in the next section. Materials used for damping are usually based on epoxies filled with small aluminium oxide particles.

4.6.1 Transducer bandwidth

Even though a transducer is specified to have a central frequency, the bandwidth of modern transducers is extremely large, as shown in Figure 4.9. For example, a transducer with a central frequency (f_0) of 3 MHz can often cover a frequency bandwidth of 1–5 MHz. This means that, rather than having to have several transducers operating at, for example 2,3,4 and 5 MHz, one can use a single transducer for many applications. As shown later in Section 4.11.2, the very wide bandwidth also means that applications in which the signal is transmitted at one frequency but

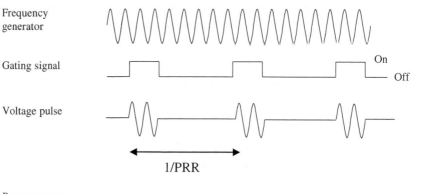

Frequency generator

Gating signal On / Off

Voltage pulse

$$1/PRR$$

Pressure wave low transducer damping

Pressure wave high transducer damping

time

Figure 4.8

Voltage pulses are applied to the face of the piezoelectric element by gating the output of a frequency generator. The pulses are produced at a certain rate, termed the pulse repetition rate (PRR). A transducer with low mechanical damping produces a pressure wave which lasts considerably longer than the driving voltage pulse. Increasing the mechanical damping (bottom row) reduces the duration of the pressure wave.

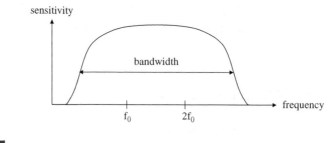

sensitivity

bandwidth

f_0 $2f_0$ frequency

Figure 4.9

Sensitivity vs. frequency for a broadband transducer. The bandwidth corresponds to the frequency range over which the sensitivity is greater than one-half of the maximum sensitivity. Note that the bandwidth can be larger than the value of f_0 itself.

received at the second harmonic frequency ($2f_0$) can be performed using a single transducer, rather than having to use two different transducers. The higher the mechanical damping, the larger is the bandwidth of the transducer. Recent developments in materials engineering have resulted in, for example, the PZT being grown as small, oriented crystals (as opposed to small particulates being embedded in a polymer matrix) and this has increased the efficiency and bandwidth of transducers. The relationship between central frequency and bandwidth is usually quantified in terms of a quality (Q) factor, defined as the ratio of the central frequency to the bandwidth. Very low values of Q ~1–2 produce very high bandwidths.

4.6.2 Beam geometry and lateral resolution

The two-dimensional beam profile from a transducer with a single flat piezoelectric crystal is shown in Figure 4.10.

The wave pattern very close to the transducer face is extremely complicated, with many areas in which the intensity falls to zero, and so this region is not useful for diagnostic scanning. This region is termed the near-field, or Fresnel, zone. Beyond this zone, the ultrasound beam does not oscillate in intensity but rather decays exponentially with distance: this is termed the far-field or Fraunhofer zone. The boundary between the two zones, termed the near-field boundary (NFB), occurs at a distance (Z_{NFB}) from the transducer face given by:

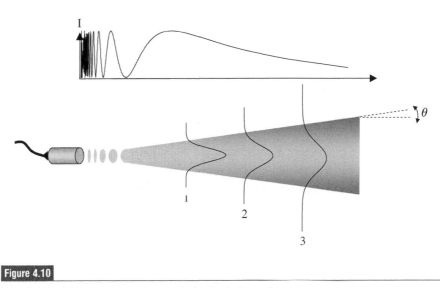

Figure 4.10

Lateral and axial beam patterns from a single element transducer.

$$Z_{NFB} \approx \frac{r^2}{\lambda},$$
(4.24)

where r is the radius of the transducer, and λ is the wavelength of the ultrasound in tissue. At the NFB, the field has a lateral beamwidth which is approximately equal to the diameter of the transducer. Beyond the NFB, the beam diverges in the lateral direction, with the angle of deviation (θ, shown in Figure 4.10) given by:

$$\theta = \arcsin\left(\frac{0.61\lambda}{r}\right).$$
(4.25)

Example 4.4 Calculate the position of the NFB for a transducer operating at 3 MHz, with a crystal diameter of 1 cm. What is the approximate beam width at a distance of 10 cm from the transducer surface?

Solution Assuming that the speed of sound in tissue is 1540 m/s, the wavelength of a 3 MHz pulse of ultrasound is $1540/(3\times10^6) = 5.13\times10^{-4}$ m ~0.05 cm. Therefore, the position of the NFB is ~(0.25/0.05) ~5 cm from the tranducer surface.
The divergent angle from Equation (4.25) is given by:

$$\theta = \arcsin\left(\frac{0.61\lambda}{r}\right) = \arcsin\left(\frac{0.61c}{rf}\right) = \arcsin\left(\frac{0.61 * 1540 \text{ms}^{-1}}{0.005\text{m} * 3 \times 10^6 \text{s}^{-1}}\right) \approx 3.6°.$$

If one assumes that the beamwidth at the NFB is 1 cm, then the beamwidth at a distance of 10 cm (5 cm from the NFB) is given by:

$$1 + 5\tan(3.6°) \approx 1.31 \text{ cm}.$$

In the far-field, Figure 4.10 shows that the lateral beam shape is approximately Gaussian. The lateral resolution is defined as the FWHM which is given by:

$$\text{FWHM} = 2.36\sigma,$$
(4.26)

where σ is the standard deviation of the Gaussian function.
It should also be noted that side-lobes are also produced by a single element transducer, with the first zero of the side-lobe present at an angle φ given by:

$$\varphi = \arcsin\left(\frac{0.61\lambda}{r}\right).$$
(4.27)

These side-lobes can introduce artifacts into an image if the lobes are back-scattered from tissue which is outside the region being studied.

4.6.3 Axial resolution

The axial resolution refers to the closest distance that two boundaries can lie in a direction parallel to the beam propagation and still be resolved as two separate features rather than as one 'combined' structure. The axial resolution has a value given by:

$$\text{Axial resolution} = \frac{1}{2}p_d c. \tag{4.28}$$

where p_d is the pulse duration (in seconds). The value of the axial resolution is therefore equal to one half the pulse length. A graphical explanation of the relationship is given in Figure 4.11, which shows a single RF pulse of three cycles being transmitted through tissue. The two different reflected signals from boundaries 1 and 2 are just resolvable (i.e. not overlapping) if the distance between the two boundaries is one-half the pulse length, as it is set to be in Figure 4.11.

Typical values of axial resolution are 1.5 mm at a frequency of 1 MHz, and 0.3 mm at 5 MHz. However, attenuation of the ultrasound beam increases at higher frequencies (1 dB cm^{-1} MHz^{-1}), and so there is a trade-off between penetration depth and axial spatial resolution. High frequency ultrasound transducers can produce very high resolution, but imaging can only be performed close to the surface. For example, frequencies of 40 MHz can be used for high resolution skin imaging, and investigating surface pathologies such as melanomas. The axial resolution can also be improved by increasing the degree of transducer damping. Finally, it should be noted that transducers with high bandwidth provide both low frequencies for better penetration, and high frequencies for better spatial resolution.

4.6.4 Transducer focusing

Since a single flat element transducer has a relatively poor lateral resolution, transducers are focused to produce a 'tighter' ultrasound beam. There are two basic methods to produce a focused transducer: either a concave lens constructed of plastic can be placed in front of the piezoelectric element, or else the face of the element itself can be manufactured as a curved surface as shown in Figure 4.7 (bottom right). The shape of the curvature is defined in terms of an f-number (f#):

$$f\# = \frac{\text{focal distance}}{\text{aperture dimension}}, \tag{4.29}$$

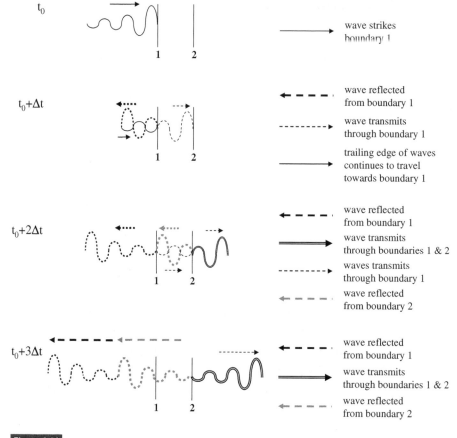

Figure 4.11

Two boundaries (1 and 2) are separated by one-half of the length of a pulse of ultrasound transmitted into the body from a transducer. The echoes from the two boundaries (bottom diagram) are just distinguishable, since they do not overlap in time. If the two boundaries were separated by a smaller distance, then the two returning echoes could not be resolved and the two boundaries would be represented by one very thick feature.

where the aperture dimension corresponds to the size of the element. The point at which the ultrasound beam is focused, i.e. at which the lateral beamwidth is most narrow, is termed the focal point and lies at a distance called the focal distance (F) away from the face of the transducer. Except for very strongly focusing transducers, with highly curved surfaces, one can approximate the focal distance to be the same as the radius of curvature of the lens or PZT element.

As is the case for a flat transducer, the lateral resolution of a focused transducer is improved the higher the operating frequency. In addition, a smaller diameter curved transducer focuses the beam to a tighter spot than a larger diameter transducer. The lateral resolution is given by $\lambda F/D$, where D is the diameter of the transducer.

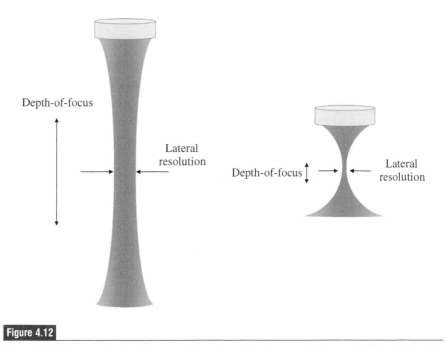

Depth-of-focus

Lateral resolution

Depth-of-focus

Lateral resolution

Figure 4.12

The trade-off between depth-of-focus and lateral resolution for a weakly-focused (left) and strongly-focused (right) single element transducer. A better lateral resolution is accompanied by a smaller depth-of-focus, and vice versa.

Choosing the focusing power of the transducer is a compromise between the highest spatial resolution and the depth over which a reasonable spatial resolution can be achieved. This is illustrated in Figure 4.12, which shows a weakly-focused transducer on the left, and a strongly-focused one on the right. The disadvantage of a strongly-focused transducer is clear: at locations away from the focal plane the beam diverges much more sharply than for the weakly-focused transducer. This is quantified via the on-axis depth-of-focus (DOF), which is defined to be the distance over which the beam intensity is at least 50% of its maximum value.

4.7 Transducer arrays

Single element arrays for imaging have been superseded by large arrays comprising many small piezoelectric elements [1]. These arrays enable two-dimensional images to be acquired by electronically steering the ultrasound beam through the patient, while the operator holds the transducer at a fixed position. Sophisticated electronics are used to produce a dynamically changing focus both during pulse transmission and signal reception, which results in high spatial resolution throughout the image. There are two basic types of array transducer, linear and phased.

4.7.1 Linear arrays

A linear array consists of a large number, typically 128–512, of rectangularly shaped piezoelectric elements. The space between elements is termed the kerf, and the distance between their centres is called the pitch, shown in Figure 4.13. Each element is unfocused, and mechanically and electrically isolated from its neighbours: mechanical isolation is achieved by filling each kerf with acoustic isolating material. The size of the pitch in a linear array ranges from $\lambda/2$ to $3\lambda/2$, where λ is the ultrasound wavelength in tissue. Overall, a linear array is usually ~1 cm in width and 10–15 cm in length: an example is shown in Figure 4.13.

The mode of operation of a linear array is shown in Figure 4.14. A small number of elements are 'excited' by separate voltage pulses to produce one beam of ultrasound entering the tissue. To provide a degree of focusing, the individual elements within this subgroup are excited at slightly different times, with the outer ones excited first and the inner ones after a certain delay. This produces a curved wavefront which focuses at an effective focal point. When all of the backscattered echoes from this ultrasound pulse have been acquired, a second beam is sent out by exciting a different subset of elements, as shown in the centre of Figure 4.14. The sequential excitation of elements is continued until all such groups have been excited. If an even number of elements is used for each subgroup, then the process can be repeated using excitation of an odd number of elements to produce focal

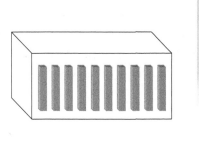
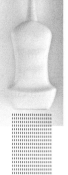
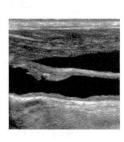

Figure 4.13

Design and operation of a linear array. (left) A large number of rectangular piezoelectric elements form a one-dimensional array. Each element is connected by a small coaxial cable to the voltage source. (centre) A commercial linear array, with the dashed lines showing the ultrasound beams that are sent out sequentially from left-to-right. (right) A two-dimensional ultrasound image acquired using a linear array.

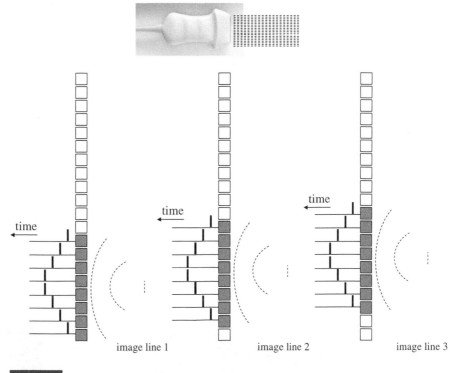

image line 1   image line 2   image line 3

Figure 4.14

Operation of a linear array. Sequential excitation of a small subgroup of the elements is used to produce a series of ultrasound lines which lie parallel to one another, and thus the image is built-up sequentially. Application of voltage pulses which are slightly delayed in time with respect to one another produces an effective focused beam for each line.

points at locations between those acquired previously. In this fashion, almost twice as many scan lines as there are transducer elements can be formed. It should be noted that, although focusing can be achieved in one-dimension, the direction perpendicular to the image plane, the so-called elevation plane, cannot be focused. Therefore, many arrays have a curved lens to produce a focus in this dimension. Linear arrays are used when a large field-of-view is required close to the surface of the array, and are a mainstay of musculoskeletal applications, for example.

4.7.2 Phased arrays

Phased arrays are much smaller than linear arrays, typically 1–3 cm in length and 1 cm wide, with fewer elements, each element being less than 1 mm in width: an example is shown on the left of Figure 4.15. Phased arrays are widely used in applications in which there is a small 'acoustic window', e.g. where there is only a small part of the body through which the ultrasound can enter without

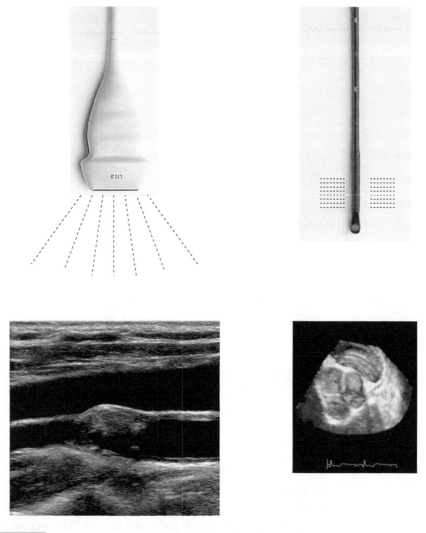

Figure 4.15

Images from (left) a conventional phased array and (right) a transoesophageal phased array.

encountering bone or air. An example is in cardiac imaging in which the ultrasound must pass between the ribs to avoid large reflections from the bone. Very small arrays can also be constructed for transoesophageal probes, which are also used in cardiac studies: an example is shown on the right of Figure 4.15.

4.7.3 Beam-forming and steering via pulse transmission for phased arrays

The basic operation of a phased array is shown in Figure 4.16. For each line in the image every element in the array is excited by voltage pulses which are applied at

time

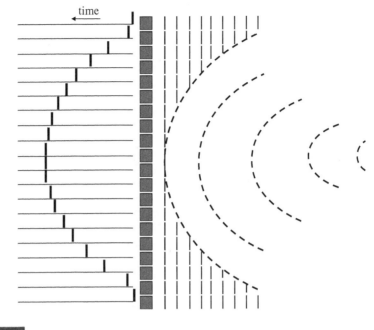

Figure 4.16

Beam-forming during ultrasound transmission. Applying voltage pulses to each individual element of the array at different times produces a composite wavefront. Applying the voltages symmetrically with respect to the centre elements, with the top and bottom elements excited first, causes the beam to focus at a point which is half-way along the array.

slightly different times. The sum of all of the individual waves from each small element makes an effective wavefront, a process known as beam-forming. In the example shown in Figure 4.16, the elements are excited symmetrically with respect to the centre of the array, and therefore produce a focal point in the tissue half-way along the length of the array.

To produce a full two-dimensional image the beam needs to be steered, and Figure 4.17 shows how, by changing the timing delays, beam-steering can be achieved.

A process termed 'dynamic focusing' or 'dynamic aperture' can be used to optimize the lateral resolution over the entire depth of tissue being imaged, as shown in Figure 4.18. Initially, using only a small number of elements produces a small focal point close to the transducer surface. At larger depths, the number of elements necessary to achieve the best lateral resolution increases. Therefore, in dynamic focusing the number of elements excited is increased dynamically during transmission. The advantage of this technique is that very high lateral resolution can be achieved throughout the entire depth of the scan. The disadvantage is that multiple scans are required to build up a single line in the B-mode image, and therefore the frame rate is reduced compared to acquiring only one single scan per line.

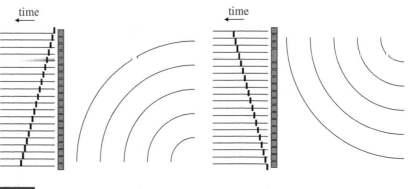

Figure 4.17

Beam steering using phased arrays. By changing the pattern of excitation of all the elements, the beam can be steered to a point below (left) and above (right) the centre of the array.

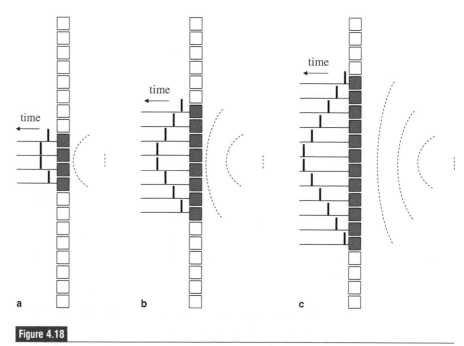

Figure 4.18

The process of dynamic focusing involves exciting an increasing number of elements in order to dynamically focus at different depths within the tissue. First, a small number of elements are used to acquire signals from very close to the transducer surface. The time required to acquire the backscattered echoes from such a shallow depth is very short, and so subsequent excitations using a larger number of elements for focusing at points deeper within tissue can be executed rapidly.

In a phased array, the length of each element defines the 'slice thickness' of the image in the elevation dimension, and is typically between 2 and 5 mm. If improved resolution is required in this dimension then, as for a linear array, a curved lens can be incorporated into the transducer.

4.7.4 Analogue and digital receiver beam-forming for phased arrays

Using a phased array transducer, the effective focal length and aperture of the transducer can also be changed dynamically while the signal is being received, a process termed 'receiver beam-forming'. This process is essentially the reverse of dynamic focusing during signal transmission covered in the previous section. During the time required for the backscattered echoes to return to the transducer, incremental delays are introduced to the voltages recorded by each element of the transducer. These delays result in each backscattered signal effectively being 'in focus', as shown in Figure 4.19.

The advent of cheap, fast digital electronics components has enabled much of the analogue circuitry to be replaced by its digital equivalent, with improvements in stability and performance. For example, the analogue receiver beam-former shown in Figure 4.19 can be replaced by a digital one simply by directly digitizing the signals with an ADC for each channel. In this design, all the data can be stored digitally, and then any chosen time delays can be introduced in post-processing to produce signals which add together perfectly coherently. There are, however, some challenges to the digital approach. For example, many more high-speed analogue-to-digital converters are needed, and these must be precisely calibrated against each other. Nevertheless, as in all of the medical imaging devices outlined in this book, integration of digital electronics into receiver design continues to improve image quality significantly.

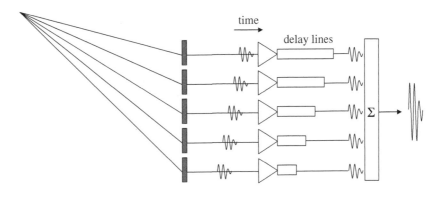

Figure 4.19

The process of receiver beam-forming. Individual echoes from the focal point reach each element in the array at slightly different times. Summation of the signals at this point would result in partially destructive interference and signal loss. After amplification, each signal is delayed by a time specified by the path length from the focal point to the transducer. After passing through the various delay lines, the signals are now in-phase and so are co-added to produce the maximum signal.

4.7.5 Time gain compensation

The summed signals from the receiver beam-former have a large range of amplitudes: very strong signals appear from, for example, reflections at fat/tissue boundaries close to the transducer, and very weak signals from soft tissue/soft tissue boundaries much deeper within the body. The total range of signal amplitudes may be as high as a factor of 100 dB. After beam-forming, the signals are passed through an amplifier to increase the signal prior to digitization. However, the amplifiers cannot provide linear gain (equal amplification) for signals with a dynamic range greater than about 40–50 dB, and so for a 100 dB dynamic range the weaker signals would be attenuated or lost completely. Therefore, a process called time-gain compensation (TGC) is used, in which the amplification factor is increased as a function of time after transmission of the ultrasound pulse. Signals arising from structures close to the transducer (early returning echoes) are amplified by a smaller factor than those from greater depths (later returning echoes). The effect of TGC is to compress the dynamic range of the backscattered echoes, as shown in Figure 4.20. The slope of the graph of amplifier gain vs. time is the TGC, which is measured in units of dB per second. TGC is under operator control and typically has a number of preset values for standard clinical imaging protocols.

The final step before digitizing the signal is rectification, i.e. to take the complex waveform and transform it into a magnitude-mode signal. This is performed via a quadrature demodulator followed by envelope detection.

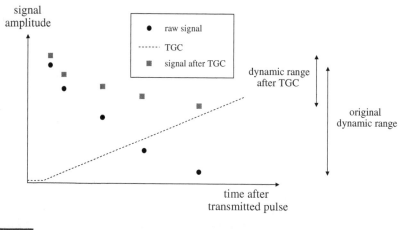

Figure 4.20

The effects of time-gain compensation in reducing the dynamic range of the signals received from close to the transducer surface and deep in tissue.

4.7.6 Multi-dimensional arrays

As outlined in previous sections, one-dimensional phased arrays can focus and steer the ultrasound beam only in the lateral dimension, with focusing in the elevation dimension requiring a lens or curved elements. Increasing the dimensionality of the array by adding extra rows of crystals allows focusing in the elevation dimension, but adds to the complexity of the transducer. If a small number of rows is added, typically three to ten, then the array is called a 1.5-dimensional array, and limited focusing in the elevation direction can be achieved. If a large number of rows is added, up to a value equal to the number of elements in each row, then this geometry constitutes a true two-dimensional array. Examples of both 1.5D and 2D arrays are shown in Figure 4.21. The two-dimensional array

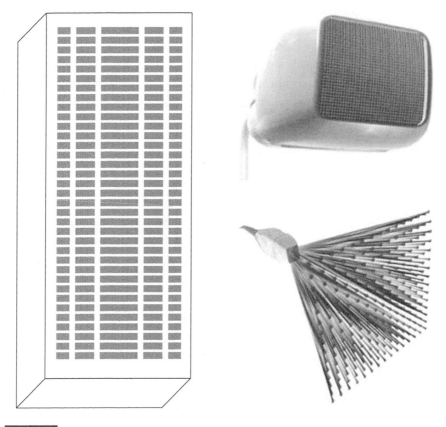

Figure 4.21

Multi-dimensional array transducers. (left) A 1.5-dimensional array, with five elements in the elevation direction which can be used to focus the beam in this dimension. (upper right) A 50 × 50 two-dimensional array transducer, which can be used for beam-forming and beam steering in two dimensions (below right).

can be used for full three-dimensional data acquisition, whereas the 1.5-D array requires mechanical movement in the third dimension. Three-dimensional imaging is playing an increasingly important role in both foetal and cardiac imaging and so larger numbers of two-dimensional arrays are now becoming commercially available.

4.7.7 Annular arrays

Linear and phased arrays are very difficult to construct at very high frequencies (> 20 MHz) and so a third type of array, the annular array, finds use at such frequencies. An annular array is shown schematically in Figure 4.22. This array is capable of two-dimensional dynamic focusing, and typically has far fewer elements (5–10) than a linear or regular phased array. Individual rings of piezoelectric material are formed and kerfs in-between the elements are filled with acoustically-isolating material. Beam-forming in both transmit and receive mode is also extremely simple. The major disadvantage of the annular array is that mechanical motion must be used to sweep the beam through tissue to form an image, but highly accurate mechanical units are produced commercially and can be integrated into the design.

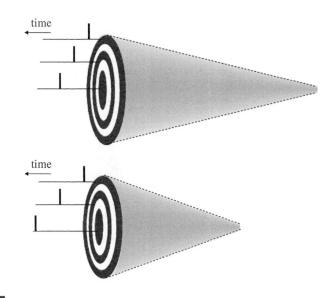

Figure 4.22

Mode of operation of an annular array. Dynamic focusing can be performed in two-dimensions simultaneously by varying the time at which each element of the array is excited. Rings of piezoelectric material (shown in black) are separated from each other by acoustic isolation material.

4.8 Clinical diagnostic scanning modes

There are three basic modes of diagnostic 'anatomical imaging' using ultrasound, A-mode, M-mode and B-mode. Depending upon the particular clinical application, one or more of these modes may be used. Recent technical advances including the use of compound imaging and three-dimensional imaging are also described in this section. The use of ultrasound to measure blood flow in covered in Section 4.10.

4.8.1 A-mode scanning: opthalmic pachymetry

An amplitude (A)-mode scan acquires a one-dimensional 'line-image' which plots the amplitude of the backscattered echo vs. time. The major application is opthalmic corneal pachymetry, which is a noninvasive technique for measuring corneal thickness. A small, high frequency (10–20 MHz) ultrasound probe is placed on the centre of the cornea after the cornea has been treated with a topical anaesthetic. Corneal pachymetry is used in chronic conditions such as glaucoma and for pre- and post-operative evaluation of corneal transplants and refractive surgery. An example of an A-mode scan is shown in Figure 4.23.

4.8.2 M-mode echocardiography

Motion (M)-mode scanning acquires a continuous series of A-mode lines and displays them as a function of time. The brightness of the displayed M-mode signal represents the amplitude of the backscattered echo. The lines are displayed with an incremental time-base on the horizontal axis, as shown in Figure 4.24.

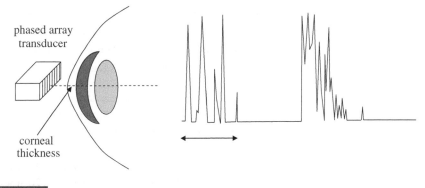

phased array
transducer

corneal
thickness

Figure 4.23

Use of A-mode ultrasound scanning to measure the corneal thickness of the eye. A single line of high frequency ultrasound is used, and the one-dimensional signal plot is shown on the right. The double-headed arrow represents the thickness of the cornea.

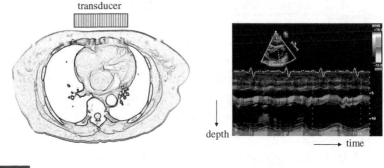

transducer

depth ⟶ time

M-mode data acquisition. The transducer is placed above the heart and sends out a single line of ultrasound. An A-mode scan is recorded, and as soon as the last echo has been acquired, the A-mode scan is repeated. The horizontal time-axis increments for each scan, and therefore a time-series of one-dimensional scans is built up. A straight line represents a structure that is stationary, whereas the front of the heart shows large changes in position.

Several thousands of lines can be acquired per second, and so real-time display of dynamic movements is possible. M-mode scanning is used most commonly in cardiac and foetal cardiac imaging.

4.8.3 Two-dimensional B-mode scanning

Brightness (B)-mode scanning is the most commonly used procedure in clinical diagnosis and produces a two-dimensional image, such as that shown in Figure 4.1, through a cross-section of tissue. Each line in the image is an A-mode line, with the intensity of each echo being represented by the brightness on the two-dimensional scan. Scanning through the body is achieved using electronic steering of the beam for linear and phased arrays, or by mechanical motion for annular arrays. As mentioned earlier, three-dimensional B-mode imaging can be performed using either a 1.5-D or 2-D phased array transducer.

Example 4.5   An image is to be acquired up to a 10 cm depth. The frame rate is set to 64 Hz, how many lines can be acquired in the image?

Solution   It takes 130 μs after transmission of the ultrasound pulse for the most distant echo to return to the transducer. If the image consists of 120 lines, then the total time to acquire one frame is 15.6 ms and the frame rate is 64 Hz. If the depth-of-view is increased, then the number of lines must be reduced to maintain the same frame rate.

4.8.4   Compound scanning

Compound scanning [2] effectively acquires an ultrasound image from multiple angles and then combines the images together. The multiple angles are achieved using a phased array with different beam forming schemes. The major advantage of compound scanning is that it reduces the degree of speckle in the image. Since the pattern of constructive and destructive interference depends upon the angle of the incident ultrasound, each separate image has a different contribution from speckle, but the same 'true' features are present in all of the views. As a result, combination of the images produces a composite image with reduced speckle. An example of compound scanning is shown in Figure 4.25. A second advantage is that, in a single view, any boundary or structure with irregular curvature which is parallel to the beam will not produce a signal. However, by using multiple angles these structures will give a signal in at least some of the views, and therefore also in the composite image: this phenomenon is also well-illustrated in Figure 4.25. Finally, artifacts such as acoustic enhancement or shadowing (Section 4.14) are reduced. Compound scanning can be integrated with Doppler scans, harmonic imaging and two-dimensional and three-dimensional imaging. The major disadvantage of compound scanning is the increased amount of time that it takes to acquire the images, meaning that a much lower frame-rate must be used.

A second mode of compound imaging is called frequency compounding. In this method, multiple frequencies rather than multiple angles are used to construct the composite image. The appearance of the speckle pattern depends upon the

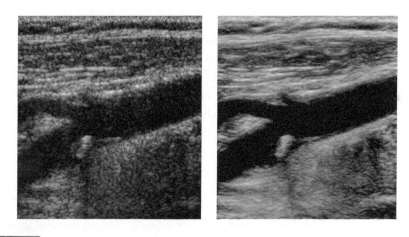

Figure 4.25

Comparison of a carotid artery bifurcation acquired using a conventional B-mode scan on the left, and a compound scan with nine different orientations on the right.

frequency, and so does not add constructively between views. The transducer must, of course, have a large enough bandwidth to cover the frequency range.

4.9 Image characteristics

The major contributing factors to signal-to-noise, spatial resolution and contrast-to-noise have already been covered, and are summarized briefly here.

4.9.1 Signal-to-noise

The signal intensity of backscattered ultrasound signals is affected by:

(i) The intensity of the ultrasound pulse transmitted by the transducer – the higher the intensity, the higher the amplitude of the detected signals. The longer the pulse, also the higher is the signal intensity. The intensity of the ultrasound pulse is limited by FDA guidelines on the amount of energy that is safe to use during a scan. This topic is further discussed in Section 4.12.

(ii) The operating frequency of the transducer – the higher the frequency, the greater the tissue attenuation, and therefore the lower the signal at large depths within the body.

(iii) The type of focusing used – the stronger the focusing at a particular point, the higher the energy per unit area of the ultrasound wave, and the higher the signal at that point. However, outside the depth-of-focus, the energy per unit area is very low, as is the image SNR.

There are two major sources of noise in ultrasound images. The first, speckle, gives a granular appearance to what should appear as a homogeneous tissue. The second contribution, termed 'clutter', corresponds to signals arising from side-lobes, grating lobes, multi-path reverberation, and tissue motion. Compound imaging can be used to reduce speckle, and harmonic imaging (covered later in Section 4.11.2) can reduce clutter.

4.9.2 Spatial resolution

(i) Lateral resolution. For a single element transducer, the higher the degree of focusing the better is the spatial resolution at the focal spot, at the cost of a reduced depth-of-focus. The higher the frequency, the better is the lateral resolution for both single element and phased array transducers.

(ii) Axial resolution. The axial resolution is given by one-half the length of the ultrasound pulse. The higher the degree of damping, or the higher the operating frequency, the shorter is the pulse and the better the axial resolution.

4.9.3 Contrast-to-noise

Factors which affect the SNR also contribute to the image CNR. Noise sources such as clutter and speckle reduce the image CNR, especially for small pathologies within tissue.

4.10 Doppler ultrasound for blood flow measurements

Non-invasive measurements of blood flow are a critical component of diagnosis in a number of pathological conditions. Ultrasound can measure blood velocity by taking advantage of the Doppler effect. This effect is familiar in everyday life as, for example, the higher frequency of an ambulance siren as it approaches than when it is driving away. The ultrasound signal from blood has its origin in signal scatter from red blood cells (RBCs), which have a diameter of ~7–10 μm. Blood flow, either towards or away from the transducer, alters the frequency of the backscattered echoes compared to the transmitted ultrasound frequency from the transducer. If blood is flowing towards the transducer the detected frequency is higher than the transmitted frequency, and vice versa. Phased array transducers can be used to localize blood flow measurements to a specified vessel, or region of a vessel, by acquiring B-mode images. From these B-mode images the vessel size can be estimated, and measured blood velocities converted into blood flow values. Blood flow measurements can be very useful in detecting vessel stenoses, and unusual blood flow patterns.

In the example shown in Figure 4.26, the direction of blood flow is towards the transducer, and therefore the effective frequency (f_i^{eff}) of the incident ultrasound beam for the moving RBCs is higher than the actual frequency transmitted (f_i):

$$f_i^{eff} = \frac{c + v \cos\theta}{\lambda} = \frac{f_i(c + v \cos\theta)}{c}. \tag{4.30}$$

The same process occurs during signal reception, and so the frequency of the ultrasound received by the transducer (f_{rec}) is given by:

$$f_{rec} = \frac{f_i^{eff}(c + v \cos\theta)}{c} = \frac{f_i(c + v \cos\theta)^2}{c^2} = f_i + \frac{2f_i v \cos\theta}{c} + \frac{f_i v^2 \cos^2\theta}{c^2}. \tag{4.31}$$

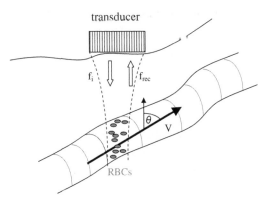

transducer

f_i f_{rec}

θ

v

RBCs

Showing the origin of the Doppler shift in ultrasound imaging of blood flow. The ultrasound beam is scattered from the RBCs in a vessel. The backscattered ultrasound beam is detected by the transducer at a slightly different frequency (f_{rec}) from that transmitted (f_i) into the body.

The overall increase in frequency, the Doppler shift (f_D), is therefore given by:

$$f_D = f_i - f_{rec} = \frac{2f_i v\cos\theta}{c} + \frac{f_i v^2 \cos^2\theta}{c^2} \approx \frac{2f_i v\cos\theta}{c}. \qquad (4.32)$$

The second term in the Doppler equation is much less than the first since $v \ll c$, and so can be ignored. From Equation (4.32), the blood velocity is given by:

$$v = \frac{cf_D}{2f_i\cos\theta}. \qquad (4.33)$$

Using values of f_i = 5 MHz, θ = 45°, and v = 50 cm s^{-1} gives a Doppler shift of 2.3 kHz. The fractional change in frequency is extremely small, in this case less than 0.05%. Doppler measurements are typically performed at a relatively high frequency, for example 5 MHz, since the intensity of the scattered signal is proportional to the fourth power of the frequency. An accurate measurement of blood velocity can only be achieved if the angle θ is known and so B-mode scans are usually acquired at the same time. A fixed error in the value of θ has the smallest effect when θ is small, and so in practice values of θ of less than 60° are used by suitable adjustment of the transducer orientation and positioning.

Ultrasound Doppler blood flow measurements can be performed either in pulsed wave or continuous wave mode, depending upon the particular application. These methods are described in the next two sections.

4.10.1 Pulsed wave Doppler measurements

The general scheme for acquiring pulsed wave Doppler scans is shown in Figure 4.27. A phased array transducer is used for both pulse transmission and signal reception. A series of ultrasound pulses, typically 128, are transmitted at a rate termed the pulse repetition rate (PRR), which is the inverse of the time (t_{rep}) between successive pulses. Based on a B-mode scan, a region-of-interest (ROI) is chosen which encompasses the vessel. The returning echoes can be localized to this region alone by a two-step process which is performed automatically by the ultrasound system under operator guidance. First, the transducer is focused within the ROI by appropriate time delays to each element of the array, as described previously. Second, by choosing the time delay after each ultrasound pulse is transmitted at which to start the data acquisition, and also the time for which the receiver is gated open, signals from tissue closer to and further away from the transducer are not recorded, and the detected signal originates only from the ROI. In terms of the parameters shown in Figure 4.27, the ROI is defined in terms of its minimum and maximum depths:

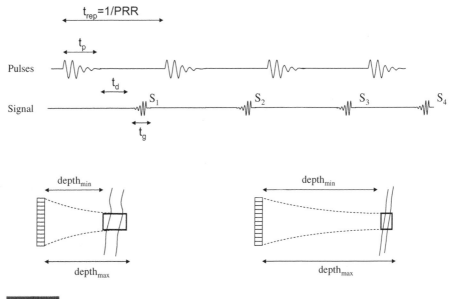

Figure 4.27

(top) General mode of operation of pulsed mode Doppler imaging. A series of signals S_1, S_2,.....S_n are acquired, and processed as shown in Figure 4.28 to estimate the blood flow. (bottom) The parameters t_p, t_g and t_d are chosen to localize the received signal to the desired ROI, defined by the focal point of the phased array transducer and the minimum and maximum required depths: shown are examples of obtaining information from a vessel close to the surface (left) and deeper within the body (right).

$$\text{depth}_{\min} = \frac{c(t_d - t_p)}{2} \quad \text{depth}_{\max} = \frac{c(t_d + t_g)}{2}. \qquad (4.34)$$

Example 4.6 An ROI has been determined to be between 7 and 9 cm deep in the tissue. At what time should the receiver be turned on after the end of pulse transmission, and for how long should the receiver be gated on? The ultrasound pulse is 5 cycles at a central frequency of 5 MHz.

Solution A train of ultrasound pulses is sent out, each pulse consisting of 5 cycles of ultrasound at a frequency of 5 MHz, resulting in a 1 μs long pulse. Assuming an ultrasound velocity of 1540 m/s in tissue, the first part of Equation (4.34) gives:

$$0.07(\text{m}) = \frac{1540(\text{ms}^{-1}) * (t_d - 1 \times 10^{-6})(\text{s})}{2},$$

from which $t_d = 92$ μs. Applying the second part of Equation (4.34):

$$0.09(\text{m}) = \frac{1540(\text{ms}^{-1}) * (92 \times 10^{-6} + t_g)(\text{s})}{2},$$

gives a gating-on time of ~25 μs.

Figure 4.28 shows the process of calculating the blood velocity within the ROI using the pulsed Doppler technique. Signals S_1, S_2.....S_n shown in Figure 4.27 each have a different phase shift with respect to the first transmitted ultrasound pulse. The amplitude of each time point within the signal is Fourier transformed to give a spectrum of the Doppler frequencies at each depth within the ROI. The frequency spectrum can then be converted into a velocity spectrum using Equation (4.32).

After the data have been processed, a 'wall-filter' is applied to the data to remove the very low frequency contributions from very slowly moving vessels or tissue walls. The data are also passed through a quadrature detector so that positive and negative Doppler frequencies can be differentiated, thus enabling the direction of flow to be determined unambiguously.

4.10.2 Duplex and triplex image acquisition

A typical Doppler image displays flow information combined with a B-mode scan. In a duplex scan the Doppler display is a colour-flow image, whereas in triplex scanning an additional Doppler spectral display is shown. A schematic Doppler

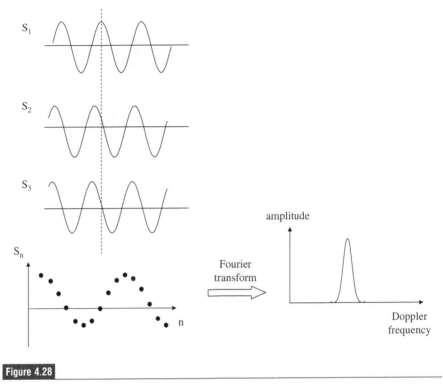

Figure 4.28

Steps in the production of a Doppler frequency distribution from one particular axial position within the ROI, determined by the particular time-point in signals $S_1 \ldots S_n$ that is analyzed. In this example a time-point is chosen at the dashed line. The signals S_1, S_2 and S_3 have slightly different phases with respect to one another due to flow. A plot of the signals (S_n), taken at the dashed line, as a function of n is shown at the bottom left. Since the value of n is directly related to the time after the initial RF pulse is applied, a Fourier transform of the S_n vs. n plot gives the Doppler frequency spectrum shown on the right. Note that there is, in general, not a single frequency but a mean value with a certain standard deviation. This process is repeated for each spatial position within the ROI.

spectral display for a chosen region within a vessel is shown in Figure 4.29. Rather than a single blood velocity, at any one instant there is a range of velocities (as shown in Figure 4.28), and this range will change significantly over the cardiac cycle, with higher velocities and a wider velocity spread typically found during systole. The Doppler spectral display plots the frequencies as a grey-scale image, with an incremental time-base along the horizontal axis providing a real-time update.

The second type of Doppler display is colour flow imaging, in which a coloured map is overlaid on top of the B-mode scan. The colour is either blue or red, representing flow towards or away from the transducer, with the intensity of the colour showing the actual velocity. These colour maps are updated in real-time along with the B-mode scans and Doppler spectral plots. The computational steps

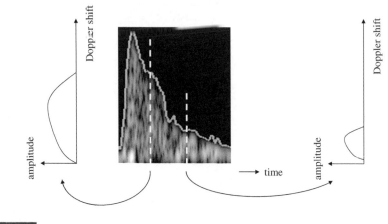

A spectral Doppler plot, with the amplitude of each frequency component of the Doppler shift being reflected in the intensity of the plot (white is the highest amplitude). The horizontal axis represents time. The left-hand plot shows high Doppler shift frequencies corresponding to high blood velocities just after the heart has reached full contraction and pumped blood into the arteries. The right-hand plot, which occurs at a later time, shows much lower Doppler shift frequencies, and coincides with the heart expanding to fill with blood ready for the next contraction.

involved in producing real time, accurate colour velocity maps are very involved, and much work has concentrated on different computationally efficient approaches [3]. At each point in the ROI determined from the B-mode scan the mean frequency is calculated and shown on the colour scale. In some systems, the mean value is displayed as the colour, with the luminance being representative of the variance. Other systems add a third colour, usually green, to indicate areas of high turbulence (detected as a large standard deviation in the flow measurement).

Although triplex imaging, as shown in Figure 4.30, provides the most information, it comes at the cost of reduced frame-rates, since all three types of measurement must be performed sequentially. Each measurement requires slightly different pulse characteristics, and so also has different image characteristics. Flow imaging requires long ultrasound pulses since the backscattered Doppler signal has a much lower intensity than the B-mode scan, whereas the B-mode scan uses short pulses to maintain high axial resolution.

4.10.3 Aliasing in pulsed wave Doppler imaging

The major limitation of pulsed-wave Doppler is that the maximum velocity that can be measured is limited by the value of the PRR, and if the velocity of the blood exceeds this value, then it will be displayed as an incorrect value which may even

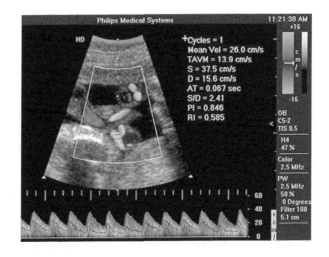

Figure 4.30

Example of a triplex scan, with greyscale B-mode, colour flow Doppler, and spectral Doppler displays of the umbilical cord.

be opposite in direction to the actual direction of flow. This phenomenon is caused by signal aliasing, as covered in Section 1.7.2, as shown in the following example.

Example 4.7 A pulsed Doppler scan is acquired with a central frequency of 5 MHz, θ value of $0°$, and a PRR of 1 kHz. There are two regions displayed which have actual blood velocities 5 cm/s and 10 cm/s. What are the phase shifts between successive signals for each region? Is there a problem with using this PRR?

Solution For the component with velocity 5 cm/s the Doppler frequency shift is:

$$f_D = \frac{2f_i v \cos\theta}{c} = \frac{2 * 5x10^6(s^{-1}) * 0.05(ms^{-1})}{1540(ms^{-1})} = 325Hz.$$

A PRR of 1 kHz corresponds to a time between signal acquisitions of 1 ms. The phase shift between successive signals is therefore:

$$\varphi(^0) = 325(s^{-1}) * 1x10^{-3}(s) * 360° = 117^0.$$

For the second component with velocity 10 cm/s the Doppler frequency shift is doubled to 650 Hz, and the phase shift to 234°. But note that a phase shift of 234° is the same as one of $-126°$. This negative phase shift corresponds to a velocity away from the transducer of 5.5 cm/s. Therefore, the area with the velocity of 10 cm/s actually appears as one with a negative velocity of 5.5 cm/s.

It is clear from the above example that signal aliasing occurs when the phase shift during each delay between successive pulses (1/PRR) is greater than 180°. Given this condition, the maximum Doppler frequency shift (f_{max}) that can be measured is:

$$f_{max} = \frac{1}{2t_{rep}} = \frac{PRR}{2}. \qquad (4.35)$$

The corresponding value of the maximum blood velocity, v_{max}, that can be measured without aliasing can be derived from Equation (4.32) setting $\cos \theta = 1$:

$$v_{max} = \frac{cf_{max}}{2f_i} = \frac{(PRR)c}{4f_i}. \qquad (4.36)$$

The value of the PRR also determines the maximum depth, d_{max}, from which flow can be measured, with a value of d_{max} given by:

$$d_{max} = \frac{ct_{rep}}{2} = \frac{c}{2PRR} = \frac{c^2}{8f_i v_{max}}. \qquad (4.37)$$

If aliasing is suspected in a pulsed-mode Doppler image, the system can be be turned either to power Doppler mode (described below) or to continuous-wave Doppler mode, described in Section 4.10.5, to confirm if this is in fact the case.

4.10.4 Power Doppler

Another potential limitation in measuring colour Doppler shifts occurs when a substantial portion of a vessel lies parallel to the face of the phased array transducer. In this case, one section of the colour velocity image shows flow towards the transducer, and the other shows flow away from the transducer. Directly below the transducer there is an area of very low signal. This effect can be removed by using the 'power Doppler' mode [4], in which the area under the magnitude of the Doppler signal is integrated to give the 'Doppler power'. In this process both positive and negative Doppler frequencies give a positive integrated power, and therefore signal voids are removed. Aliasing artifacts at high flow rates are also eliminated since the integral of an aliased signal is the same as that of a non-aliased signal. The major disadvantage with power Doppler is the loss of directional information.

4.10.5 Continuous wave Doppler measurements

CW Doppler measurements can be used when there is no need to localize exactly the source of the Doppler shifts. Many modern ultrasound systems can acquire both CW and PW Doppler data using the same phased array transducer. In CW mode the array is 'split' into two sections, one which transmits a continuous pulse of ultrasound, and the other which receives the backscattered signals. The area in which blood flow is detected is defined by the overlap of the areas defined by the transmission and reception beam-forming settings. The measured blood velocity is the average value over the entire sensitive region. In order to determine the direction of flow (towards or away from the transducer) a quadrature detector must be used. The main advantages of CW Doppler over PW Doppler methods is that the method is neither limited to a maximum depth, nor to a maximum measurable velocity. As with PW Doppler, a triplex display showing a CW Doppler image, Doppler spectral plot and B-mode scan is commonly used in diagnostic scans.

4.11 Ultrasound contrast agents

Contrast agents for ultrasound imaging comprise different types and formulations of microbubbles or microspheres [5], and are used primarily for echocardiography and Doppler imaging. In cardiac imaging they can be used for ventricular opacification, the assessment of left ventricular volume, systolic function, and delineation of the endocardial structures. By enhancing the signal intensity of Doppler ultrasound, they also make possible measurements of blood perfusion in the heart and other organs such as the liver.

4.11.1 Microbubbles

Currently there are two ultrasound agents, SonoVue and Optison, approved for worldwide clinical use. SonoVue is a microbubble which is coated with phospholipid monolayers and contains sulphur hexafluoride gas. Optison consists of microbubbles which contain perfluoropropane gas within a cross-linked serum albumen microsphere. The shells of these microbubbles are a few tens of nanometres thick, the bubble diameter being between 2 and 10 μm, see Figure 4.31. These microspheres are packaged as freeze-dried powders which can be rehydrated in physiological saline solution just before they are to be injected into the patient's bloodstream. There are many other types of microbubble in the late stages of clinical testing, with the main differences being in the particular gaseous core and exact make-up of the microbubble shell. The reason for needing an outer shell, rather than simply using a bubble of gas, is that there is a very high surface tension at the boundary between the microbubble and surrounding liquid: without the

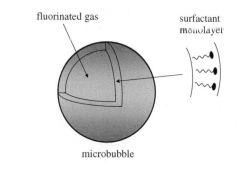

fluorinated gas   surfactant
                         monolayer

microbubble

Figure 4.31

A microbubble-based ultrasound contrast agent. The diameter of the microbubble is between 2 and 10 μm. The polymer coating is a few tens of nanometres thick.

coating, the bubbles would dissolve almost instantaneously after injection into the bloodstream.

Although it is easy to see that the characteristic impedance of a gas-filled microbubble is much different from the surrounding tissue or blood, this is not the principal reason why such agents are so effective. Since the microbubbles are filled with a compressible gas, they respond to the propagating ultrasound beam by compressing (during high pressure periods) and expanding (during low pressure periods) as shown in Figure 4.32. This means that they absorb much more energy during compression than would, for example, a relatively incompressible equivalently-sized cell in tissue. This absorbed energy is then re-radiated during expansion, resulting in a strong echo signal returning to the transducer. There is a 'resonance' condition which corresponds to the ultrasound frequency at which the degree of expansion and contraction of the bubble is greatest: this frequency is determined by the size of the microbubble, as well as the stiffness and thickness of the polymeric coating. Somewhat fortuitously, the required size for microbubbles to pass through the human capillaries (< 6–7 μm) corresponds to a resonance frequency within the diagnostic imaging frequency range.

If the ultrasound pressure wave has a high enough intensity, the linear response shown in Figure 4.32 is replaced by a non-linear one. This behaviour is due to effects such as the speed of propagation being greater when the bubble is compressed than when it expands, and also to the fact that the microbubble may distort from a perfect spherical shape during expansion. The important result is that the pressure wave which is radiated by the microbubble during expansion is also non-linear in that it contains not only components at the frequency of the transmitted ultrasound, but also significant contributions at higher harmonics of this frequency, as shown in Figure 4.33.

The presence of harmonics makes it possible to distinguish between the ultrasound pressure waves that are backscattered from the microbubbles and those from

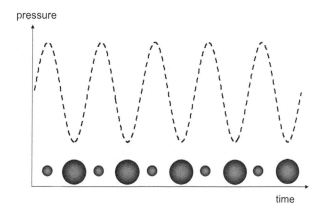

Figure 4.32

Change in the shape of a microbubble as an ultrasound pressure wave passes through the tissue in which the microbubble is located.

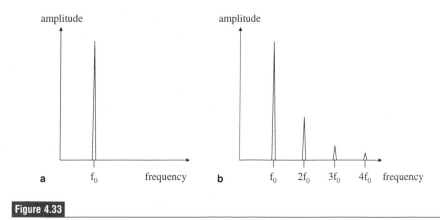

Figure 4.33

(a) Frequency spectrum of the ultrasound field backscattered from a microbubble when the incident pressure field has a low enough intensity to produce only linear effects of expansion and contraction of the microbubble. (b) If the incident pressure field is much higher, non-linear effects produce harmonics of the base frequency.

the surrounding tissue. As can be seen from Figure 4.33, the signal at $2f_0$ is the strongest harmonic and so is the most commonly used. Needless to say, the bandwidth of the transducer should be large enough so that it can efficiently transmit pulses at f_0 and also efficiently detect the signal at $2f_0$.

An extreme version of nonlinear behaviour occurs if the intensity of the incident ultrasound is high enough to destroy the microbubble. This produces a very strong backscattered signal and can be used to increase the signal in Doppler imaging, for example. In this case, the normal Doppler demodulated frequency, Δf, is multiplied by the particular harmonic that is produced and detected:

$$\Delta f_{Doppler} = \frac{nf_0 v}{c} \cos \theta, \qquad (4.38)$$

where n is the order of the harmonic. A high-pass filter is used to remove contributions from the fundamental ($n = 1$) harmonic, so that only signals from the microbubble destruction are detected. The intensity of the transmitted ultrasound pulse can be determined from the mechanical index (MI), which is a measure of the acoustic output of the particular ultrasound system. The MI is typically displayed on the ultrasound operating console, and its value can be used to control whether linear, nonlinear or destructive effects are produced during the ultrasound scan. Safety aspects of the MI are covered in Section 4.12.

4.11.2   Harmonic and pulse inversion imaging

Although it is technically possible in contrast agent imaging to detect separately the signals centred at f_0 and its harmonic at $2f_0$ using high-pass and low-pass filters, in practice there is considerable signal contamination between the two very broad frequency distributions. Pulse inversion imaging is a technique which was designed to overcome some of the limitations of second harmonic imaging [6]. Two sets of scans are acquired, as shown in Figure 4.34, with the phase of the transmitted ultrasound pulse differing by 180° in the two scans. Linear backscattering from tissue results in two signals which differ in phase by 180° in the two scans, and so addition of the two scans results in signal cancellation. However, for nonlinear scattering, the signals do not completely cancel out, with the residual signal being proportional to the degree of nonlinearity.

Second harmonic imaging has an increased lateral resolution over images at the fundamental frequency due to the higher frequency and therefore smaller

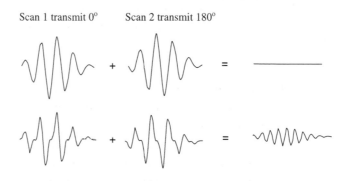

Figure 4.34

The principle of pulse inversion imaging. At the top, any signal which contains only components at f_0 is cancelled out by addition of the two scans. At the bottom, the signal contains components at both f_0 and $2f_0$: in the summed signal, the component at $2f_0$ remains.

wavelength. Also there is a reduction in what is termed ultrasound 'clutter', which refers to effects such as reverberation and reflected signal from side-lobes, since these effects do not give rise to a second harmonic signal. The only disadvantage of pulse inversion imaging is that the scan takes twice as long, or alternatively that the frame-rate is halved compared to conventional imaging.

It should be noted that in addition to using harmonic imaging in combination with contrast agents there is increasing use of 'native' second harmonic imaging in normal tissue without using contrast agents. Although the second harmonic signal is much weaker than the fundamental frequency, since for conventional power levels there are relatively minor nonlinear effects, the facts that clutter is much reduced and that lateral resolution is enhanced makes harmonic imaging a useful option in certain applications.

4.12 Safety guidelines in ultrasound imaging

Under normal scanning protocols for diagnostic radiology and cardiology, ultrasound imaging is extremely safe, with very low power levels causing insignificant increases in tissue temperature. However, there is constant monitoring of imaging protocols by various scientific and government bodies, particularly with the increased use of power-intensive scanning modes such as combined compound scanning/three-dimensional imaging/power Doppler, for example. In addition, use of microbubble contrast agents, and the correspondingly higher ultrasound powers needed to induce significant nonlinear behaviour (often culminating in bubble destruction), also increase the amount of energy deposited into the body well beyond the normal B-mode scanning conditions. There are several measures of the ultrasound energy, summarized below [7], which are used to form guidelines for different diagnostic protocols:

(i) Spatial average (SA)	Takes into account the Gaussian shape of the lateral beamwidth and calculates the average value of the Gaussian function
(ii) Temporal average (TA)	Multiplies the average intensity during the pulse by the duty cycle (the percentage of the total imaging time for which the driving voltage is gated on)
(iii) Spatial peak (SP)	Measures the peak intensity at the focal spot of the beam
(iv) Temporal peak (TP)	Measures the highest instantaneous intensity of the beam

Common acronyms used for reporting ultrasound intensities for different procedures use a combination of these terms, for example spatial average temporal average (SATA), spatial peak temporal average (SPTA), spatial peak pulse average (SPPA), spatial peak temporal peak (SPTP), spatial peak (SP) and spatial average (SA).

Tissue heating and cavitation are the two mechanisms by which destructive bioeffects can potentially occur during an ultrasound scan. For tissue heating, the intensity of the ultrasound beam and the duration of the scan are both important parameters. For cavitation, the relevant parameter is the pulse peak rarefactional pressure amplitude, which in Doppler ultrasound can be between ~0.7 and 3.5 Mpa. This is particularly relevant to gas echo-contrast agents, in which cavitation of the bubbles can occur. The acoustic output from ultrasound medical devices is directly regulated only in the USA. There is an overall maximum limit of 720 mW/cm^2 for the derated I_{SPTA}. If the systems have a real-time output display standard (ODS) of safety indices such as mechanical index (MI) and thermal index (TI), then the FDA limits (referred to as track 1) are lifted, and much higher intensities can be used (referred to as track 3), as shown in Table 4.2. The thermal index is determined as the ratio of the total acoustic power to that required to produce a maximum temperature increase of 1 °C. There are three TI values, TIS (TI soft tissue), TIB (bone) and TIC (cranial bone). The mechanical index is mathematically defined as:

$$MI = \frac{max\left[p_r(z)e^{-0.0345f_0z}\right]}{\sqrt{f_0}}, \qquad (4.39)$$

where p_r is the axial value of the rarefactional pressure measured in water.

The TI and MI are only rough approximations of the risk of inducing biological effects, with values less than 1 indicating safe operation. For B-mode scanning, the MI is displayed, for Doppler, M-mode or colour flow imaging the TI is displayed. The FDA has an upper limit of 1.9 on the MI (0.23 for opthalmic scans). The aim of the MI is to predict the likelihood of cavitation, where the peak pressure is the critical parameter. The TI estimates the potential for producing thermally-induced

Table 4.2: Intensity limits, I_{SPTA}, (mW/cm^2)

	FDA (track 1)	ODS (track 3)
Peripheral vessel	720	720
Cardiac	430	720
Foetal, neonatal	94	720
Opthalmic	17	50

biological effects in soft tissue and bone. Both TI and MI values provide indicators of risk rather than quantifiable values.

In general, B-mode imaging is not capable of causing harmful temperature rises. Doppler scans can potentially produce harmful temperature increases, particularly at bone/soft-tissue interfaces since longer pulses and higher pulse-repetition rates in Doppler imaging compared to B-mode imaging result in higher average intensities. In addition, in pulsed Doppler the beam is focused into a relatively small volume and kept stationary. A diagnostic procedure that produces a maximum temperature rise of no more than 1.5°C above normal physiological levels is allowed clinically. Any procedure that elevates embryonic and foetal *in situ* temperature above 41 °C for five minutes or more is considered potentially hazardous.

4.13 Clinical applications of ultrasound

Ultrasound finds very wide use in radiology, due to its relatively low-cost, high portability, and noninvasive nature. Recent developments such as compound scanning, harmonic imaging and two-dimensional arrays have increased the quality and utility of ultrasound significantly. Ultrasound is the only modality able to provide very high frame-rate real-time imaging over significant periods. It has almost no contraindications, unlike MRI which cannot be used for patients with many types of implant, and uses no ionizing radiation. It is also the only modality that is routinely used during pregnancy. As examples, applications to obstetrics, breast imaging, musculoskeletal damage and cardiac studies are outlined briefly below.

4.13.1 Obstetrics and gynaecology

Parameters such as the size of the foetal head and extent of the developing brain ventricles (for diagnosis of hydrocephalus), and the condition of the spine are measured to assess the health of the foetus. If amniocentesis is necessary to detect disorders such as Down's syndrome, then ultrasound is used for needle guidance. Doppler ultrasound is also used to measure foetal cardiac parameters such as blood velocity. Three-dimensional ultrasound provides high resolution images of the developing foetus, although such images tend to be more for show than for actual clinical diagnosis. The high spatial resolution and excellent image contrast possible are shown in Figure 4.35.

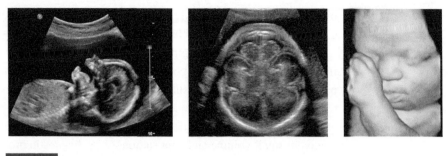

Figure 4.35

Two-dimensional B-mode scans of (left) 19 week fetus in the womb, and (centre) foetal brain. (right) Three dimensional foetal image using a two-dimensional array and mechanical steering.

4.13.2 Breast imaging

Ultrasound imaging is used to differentiate between solid and cystic lesions, and for the evaluations of lesions in young women with dense breast tissue or who are pregnant, since X-rays are not effective or not allowed, respectively [8]. Five different categories of lesion are defined by the American College of Radiography based on well-defined morphometric measures and image characteristics. High frequency ultrasound, between 9 and 12 MHz, is used for optimal image contrast, as well as for the highest axial and lateral resolution. The standard procedure is to use two-dimensional B-mode scanning. Breast lesions are generally hypoechoic, appearing darker than the surrounding tissue. Harmonic and compound imaging have recently been used extensively since they reduce the contribution from speckle, reverberation and internal-echo artifacts. In many cases, solid breast tumours are better delineated using harmonic imaging. However, due to the higher frequency of the returning echoes, B-mode scanning may be preferred for deep lesions. Two examples of breast masses detected using ultrasound are shown in Figure 4.36. Colour Doppler imaging is sometimes added to the scanning protocol, since malignancies often have higher vascularity than benign lesions. In addition to radiological diagnosis, real-time two-dimensional scanning is an effective method for image-guided needle biopsy of a lesion, in which a sample of the lesion is extracted for biochemical analysis to determine whether it is cancerous or not.

4.13.3 Musculoskeletal structure

The newer technologies of compound and harmonic scanning have made significant improvements to musculoskeletal (MSK) ultrasound imaging [9]. In particular, compound scanning improves the quality of tendon and nerve images, since

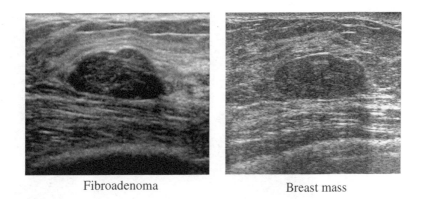

Fibroadenoma   Breast mass

Figure 4.36

(left) A fibroadenoma and (right) a breast mass, both easily visible on a two-dimensional B-mode scan.

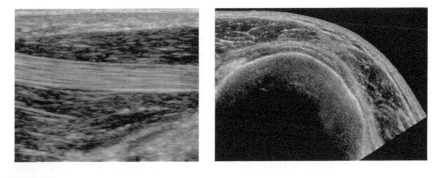

Figure 4.37

(left) Compound scan of the flexor pollicus tendon in the hand. (right) Compound scan of a rotator cuff injury in the shoulder.

these typically produce a lot of speckle. Example images are shown in Figure 4.37. Small lesions detection is also significantly improved by compound scanning. Doppler imaging can detect reduced flow in superficial vessels in diseases such as rheumatism, and other inflammatory conditions. Three-dimensional imaging is often used for imaging complicated joints. Finally, ultrasound guidance is often used for interventional MSK procedures in which needles must be placed precisely within the particular joint.

4.13.4 Echocardiography

Two-dimensional B-mode imaging of the heart is used to determine clinically-relevant parameters such as ventricular size and function [10]. Specific

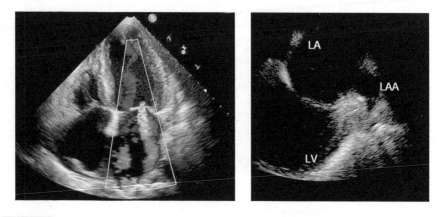

(left) Mitral regurgitation shown by colour pulsed Doppler. (right) Left atrial appendage (LAA), left ventricle (LV) and left anterior (LA) chamber.

applications are early signs of cardiac disease, such as chest pain, suspected cardiac embolisms and infarctions, valve disease and cardiac arrhythmias. The sensitivity to infarction is very high, typically a negative predictive value of ~95% after reported cases of chest pain. In addition to morphometrical measurements, echocardiography equipment is used for colour Doppler imaging for wall motion analysis, as shown in Figure 4.38, as well as being able to produce maps of myocardial strain. Similarly to nuclear medicine stress tests, stress echocardiography can also be performed after strenuous exercise. Three-dimensional ultrasound is likely to play an increasingly important role in echocardiography, due to the much higher reproducibility of quantitative measures such as ejection fraction and left ventricular mass. Microbubble contrast agents can be used to 'opacify' the left ventricle, and also to measure myocardial perfusion, but these procedures are currently not widely performed. As with many other ultrasound applications, echocardiography is a low-risk first choice scan, which does not have a large radiation dose associated with it, and can be used on patients with pacemakers, defribrillators, and stents which are MRI-incompatible. Simple portable echocardiography units are available, as are dedicated systems which incorporate pulsed-mode and continuous-wave Doppler, pulse-inversion harmonic imaging, compound scanning, three-dimensional imaging, M-mode imaging and sophisticated phased arrays.

4.14 Artifacts in ultrasound imaging

As outlined in Section 1.8, the term image artifact refers to any features in the image which do not correspond to actual tissue structures, but rather to 'errors'

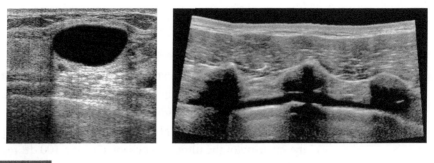

Figure 4.39.

Image artifacts caused by (left) acoustic enhancement, and (right) acoustic shadowing.

introduced by the imaging technique or instrumentation. Such artifacts must be recognized to avoid incorrect image interpretation, but once recognized can in fact give useful diagnostic information. The main artifact in ultrasound imaging, namely speckle, has already been described. It arises from the constructive and destructive interference of ultrasound scattered from very small structures within tissue, and this complicated wave pattern gives rise to high and low intensities within the tissue which are not correlated directly with any particular structure.

There are several other artifacts that appear in ultrasound images. Reverberations occur if there is a very strong reflector close to the transducer surface. Multiple reflections occur between the surface of the transducer and the reflector, and these reflections appear as a series of repeating lines in the image. These artifacts are relatively simple to detect due to the equidistant nature of the lines. Typically, they occur when the ultrasound beam encounters regions of either bone or air. Acoustic enhancement occurs when there is an area of low attenuation relative to the surrounding tissue, and therefore structures lying deeper and in-line with this area show an artificially high signal intensity. Areas which contain a high proportion of water such as cysts can show this effect. The opposite phenomenon, termed acoustic shadowing, occurs when a highly attenuating medium results in a dark area deeper below the highly attenuating medium. Solid tumours are one example of tissues which cause acoustic shadowing. Examples of acoustic enhancement and shadowing are shown in Figure 4.39.

Exercises

Reflection, transmission, refraction and scattering

4.1 Calculate the intensity transmission coefficient, T_I, for the following interfaces, assuming that the ultrasound beam is exactly perpendicular to the interface:

(i) muscle/kidney,
(ii) air/muscle, and
(iii) bone/muscle.

Discuss briefly the implications of these values of TI for ultrasound imaging.

4.2 Repeat the calculations in Exercise 4.1 with the angle of incidence of the ultrasound beam now being 45°.

4.3 Within tissue lies a strongly reflecting boundary, which backscatters 70% of the intensity of the ultrasound beam. Given a 100 dB receiver dynamic range, and an operating frequency of 3 MHz, what is the maximum depth within tissue at which this boundary can be detected?

Absorption and attenuation of ultrasound energy

4.4 Calculate the distance at which the intensity of a 1 MHz and 5 MHz ultrasound beam will be reduced by half traveling through (a) bone, (b) air, and (c) muscle.

4.5 Explain why a very fast or very slow tissue relaxation time results in a very small amount of energy being lost due to absorption.

4.6 Plot the attenuation of the ultrasound beam for 1, 5 and 10 MHz at depths within tissue of 1 cm, 5 cm, and 10 cm. For each depth calculate the fractional decrease in transmitted power, and the absolute power assuming an output power from the transducer of 100 mW/cm^2.

Single element transducers

4.7 In order to improve the efficiency of a given transducer, the amount of energy reflected by the skin directly under the transducer must be minimized. A layer of material with an acoustic impedance $Z_{matching\ layer}$ is placed between the transducer and the skin. If the acoustic impedance of the skin is denoted by Z_{skin}, and that of the transducer crystal Z_{PZT}, show mathematically that the value of $Z_{matching\ layer}$ which minimizes the energy of the reflected wave is given by:

$$Z_{matching\ layer} = \sqrt{Z_{PZT}Z_{skin}}.$$

4.8 Given values of Z_{PZT} and Z_{skin} of 30×10^5 g cm^{-2} s^{-1} and 1.7×10^5 g cm^{-2} s^{-1}, respectively, calculate what fraction of the energy from the transducer is actually transmitted into the patient.

4.9 If two matching layers are used instead of one, and the respective acoustic impedances are given by the analogues of the equation above, then calculate the increase in efficiency in transmitting power into the patient.

4.10 Consider a transducer which has a thickness given by Equation (4.22). A matching layer is used to maximize the energy transferred from the transducer to the body. Show that the thickness of this matching layer should be one-quarter of the ultrasound wavelength.

4.11 Why is the thickness of the PZT element set to one-half wavelength?

4.12 For a concave lens to focus a beam, should the speed of sound in the lens be greater than or less than in tissue?

4.13 How does the frequency profile of the ultrasound beam change as it passes through tissue? How does this affect the lateral resolution?

4.14 Consider a focused transducer with a radius of curvature of 10 cm and a diameter of 4 cm. This transducer operates at a frequency of 3.5 MHz, and transmits a pulse of duration 0.857 μs. What is the axial and lateral resolution at the focal point of the transducer?

4.15 If the axial and lateral resolution were to be improved by a factor of 2 from those calculated in Exercise 4.14, what physical or operating parameters could be changed?

4.16 Plot the transmitted frequency spectrum of an ultrasound beam from a transducer operating at a central frequency of 1.5 MHz. Assume that the transducer is damped. Repeat the plot for the beam returning to the transducer after having passed through tissue and been backscattered.

4.17 Draw the corresponding beam pattern to that shown in Figure 4.10 for a transducer operating at double the frequency. Note all of the frequency-dependent changes in the beam pattern.

Transducer arrays

4.18 Show the required timing for simultaneous steering and dynamic focusing of a phased array. For simplicity, sketch the general scheme using a small number (for example five) of elements.

4.19 Sketch the corresponding delays required for dynamic beam-forming during signal reception.

Clinical scanning modes

4.20 Use the following data to sketch the A-mode scan from Figure 4.40(a). The amplitude axis should be on a dB scale, and the time axis in microseconds. Ignore any reflected signal from the transducer/fat interface, and assume that a signal of 0 dB enters the body. At a transducer frequency of 5 MHz, the linear attenuation coefficient for muscle and liver is 5 dB cm^{-1}, and for fat is 7 dB cm^{-1}. Relevant values of the characteristic acoustic impedance and speed of sound can be found in Table 4.1.

4.21 Determine and sketch the A-mode scan using the same parameters as above, but with a time gain compensation of 0.8 dB μs^{-1}.

4.22 For the object shown in Figure 4.40(b), qualitatively sketch the B-mode ultrasound image. Ignore speckle or scatter and only consider signals

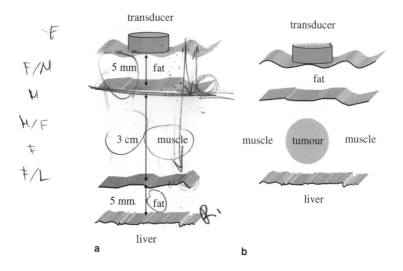

·F

F/M

M

M/F

F

F/L

a   b

Figure 4.40

See Exercises 4.20, 4.21 and 4.22.

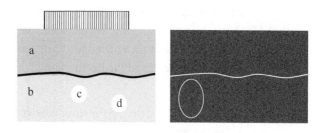

Figure 4.41

See Exercise 4.24.

backscattered from the tissue boundaries. Acoustic impedances: muscle 1.61, tumour 1.52 (x 10^5 g/cm^{2}s). Attenuation coefficients: muscle 1.0, tumour 0.4 (dB/cm/MHz). Speeds of sound: muscle 1540, tumour 750 (m/s).

4.23 In a particular real-time imaging application the transducer moves through a 90° sector with a frame rate of 30 frames per second, acquiring 128 lines of data per frame. If the image is acquired up to a depth of 20 cm, and the lateral resolution of the beam width at this depth is 5 mm, calculate the effect of transducer motion on overall image blurring, i.e. is it the dominant factor?

4.24 A B-mode scan is taken of the object in Figure 4.41 with a linear array. There are four tissue components, A and B with a boundary in-between and two spherical tumors C and D. Given the corresponding ultrasound image shown on the right what can you deduce about the acoustic characteristics of components A, B, C and D?

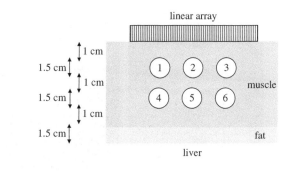

Figure 4.42

See Exercise 4.25.

Tissue	Z (x 10⁵)	c (m/s)	μ (dB/cm)
Muscle	1.7	1540	1
Fat	1.4	1450	1.7
Liver	1.6	1570	1.5
Tumour 1	1.7	1540	1
Tumour 2	1.9	3080	1
Tumour 3	10	1540	5
Tumour 4	1.9	1540	20
Tumour 5	1.9	770	1
Tumour 6	1.9	1540	1

4.25 Given the ultrasound data in the table below, sketch the B-mode scan that would be obtained from the linear sequential array in Figure 4.42 (a quantitative analysis is NOT needed, ignore any refraction of the ultrasound beam).

4.26 The three ultrasound images in Figure 4.43 are of the same object. Explain which operating parameter changes from image (a) to image (b) to image (c).

Doppler ultrasound

4.27 Sketch the Doppler spectral patterns at points 1, 2, and 3 in the stenotic artery shown in Figure 4.44 (a).

4.28 On the same scale as for Exercise 4.27, sketch the Doppler spectral plots for the situation in Figure 4.44 (b) in which the angle between the artery and the phased array transducer is altered.

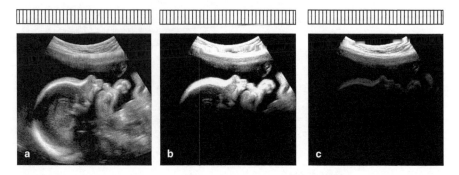

Figure 4.43

See Exercise 4.26.

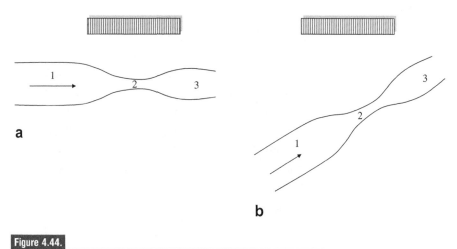

Figure 4.44.

See Exercises 4.27 and 4.28.

4.29 Show that the effects of a fixed error in the estimated angle between the transducer and the direction of flow in Doppler imaging are minimized by using a small value of the angle.

Artifacts in ultrasound imaging

4.30 Sketch the shape of the acoustic shadowing artifact produced from compound scanning.

4.31 The well-known reverberation artifact occurs when a strongly reflecting boundary within tissue is close to the transducer. Assume that there is a 2 cm thickness of muscle in front of the ribs. $Z_{crystal}$ is 33×10^5, Z_{muscle} is 1.7×10^5 and Z_{bone} is 7.8×10^5 g cm^{-2} s^{-1}, the speed of sound in muscle is 1540 m/s, and the attenuation coefficient of muscle is 1 dB/cm, calculate the time gain compensation (units of dB/microsecond) that must be used to make the intensity of each of the reverberation signals the same.

References

[1] Shung KK. The principle of multi-dimensional arrays. *Eur J Echocardiogr* 2002 Jun;**3**(2), 149–53.

[2] Jespersen SK, Wilhjelm JE and Sillesen H. Multi-angle compound imaging. *Ultrason Imaging* 1998Apr;**20**(2), 81–102.

[3] Jensen JA. *Estimation of Blood Velocities Using Ultrasound.* Cambridge: Cambridge University Press, 1996.

[4] Rubin JM, Bude RO, Carson PL, Bree RL and Adler RS. Power Doppler US: a potentially useful alternative to mean frequency-based color Doppler US. *Radiology* 1994:**190**(3), 853–6.

[5] Stride E. Physical principles of microbubbles for ultrasound imaging and therapy. *Cerebrovasc Dis* 2009;**27** Suppl. 2, 1–13.

[6] Kollmann C. New sonographic techniques for harmonic imaging – underlying physical principles. *Eur J Radiol* 2007Nov;**64**(2), 164–72.

[7] Barnett SB, Ter Haar GR, Ziskin MC *et al.* International recommendations and guidelines for the safe use of diagnostic ultrasound in medicine. *Ultrasound Med Biol* 2000;**26**(3), 355–66.

[8] Athanasiou A, Tardivon A, Ollivier L *et al.* How to optimize breast ultrasound. *European Journal of Radiology* 2009;**69**(1), 6–13.

[9] Klauser AS and Peetrons P. Developments in musculoskeletal ultrasound and clinical applications. *Skeletal Radiol* 2009Sep;**3**.

[10] Marwick TH. The future of echocardiography. *Eur J Echocardiogr* 2009Jul;**10**(5), 594–601.

5 Magnetic resonance imaging (MRI)

5.1 Introduction

Of the four major clinical imaging modalities, magnetic resonance imaging (MRI) is the one developed most recently. The first images were acquired in 1973 by Paul Lauterbur, who shared the Nobel Prize for Medicine in 2003 with Peter Mansfield for their shared contribution to the invention and development of MRI. Over 10 million MRI scans are prescribed ever year, and there are more than 4000 scanners currently operational in 2010.

MRI provides a spatial map of the hydrogen nuclei (water and lipid) in different tissues. The image intensity depends upon the number of protons in any spatial location, as well as physical properties of the tissue such as viscosity, stiffness and protein content. In comparison to other imaging modalities, the main advantages of MRI are: (i) no ionizing radiation is required, (ii) the images can be acquired in any two- or three-dimensional plane, (iii) there is excellent soft-tissue contrast, (iv) a spatial resolution of the order of 1 mm or less can be readily achieved, and (v) images are produced with negligible penetration effects. Pathologies in all parts of the body can be diagnosed, with neurological, cardiological, hepatic, nephrological and musculoskeletal applications all being widely used in the clinic. In addition to anatomical information, MR images can be made sensitive to blood flow (angiography) and blood perfusion, water diffusion, and localized functional brain activation. The main disadvantages of MRI are: (i) MR image acquisition is much slower than CT and ultrasound, and is comparable to PET: a typical clinical protocol might last 30–40 minutes with several different types of scan being run, each having a slightly different contrast, with each scan taking between five and ten minutes, (ii) a significant percentage of patients are precluded from MRI scans due to metallic implants from previous surgeries, and (iii) systems are much more expensive than CT or ultrasound units.

The MRI system comprises three major hardware components: a superconducting magnet, a set of three magnetic field gradient coils, and a radiofrequency transmitter and receiver. The superconducting magnet typically has a strength of 3 Tesla, approximately 60 000 times greater than the earth's magnetic field. This magnetic

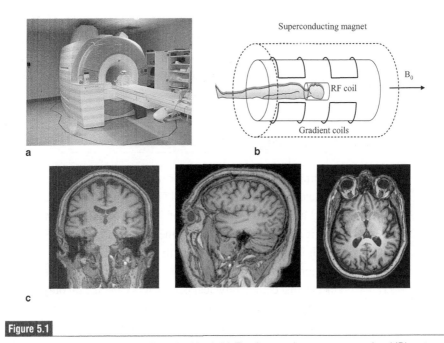

Figure 5.1

(a) A high-field clinical magnet with patient bed. (b) The three major components of an MRI system, including the superconducting magnet which produces a strong magnetic field (B_0) in the horizontal direction. Only one of the three gradient coils is shown for clarity. (c) MR images can be acquired in any orientation, shown here are coronal, sagittal and axial images, respectively, of the brain.

field causes the protons to precess at a frequency proportional to the strength of the magnetic field, i.e. there is a 'resonance' frequency. The magnetic field gradients make this resonance frequency dependent upon the spatial location of each proton in the body, thus enabling an image to be formed. A tuned radiofrequency coil transmits energy into the body at ~128 MHz for a 3 Tesla magnet, and the MRI signal is induced in the same or other RF coils which are placed close to the body.

Figure 5.1 shows a simplified schematic of the components of an MRI system, as well as a photograph of a commercial high-field scanner together with patient bed. Figure 5.1(c) shows typical brain MRI scans in three different orientations. There is excellent contrast between the grey and white matter of the brain, with the protons in lipid seen as a bright signal outside the skull. Protons in very rigid structures such as bone are normally not visible using MRI: this is evident by the thin dark line between the lipid layer and brain surface in Figure 5.1(c).

5.2 Effects of a strong magnetic field on protons in the body

In an MRI scanner the patient lies on a patient bed which slides into a very strong magnet. A typical value of the magnetic field, B_0, is 3 Tesla (30 000 Gauss), roughly

60 000 times greater than the earth's magnetic field of ~50 μT (0.5 Gauss). Numerous studies have shown no detrimental effect of such a high magnetic field, but patients must undergo a thorough check to ensure that they have no magnetic metal implants or surgical clips. The effect of placing the body in a strong magnetic field is covered in the following two sections.

5.2.1 Proton energy levels

In clinical MRI the image is formed by the signals from protons (hydrogen nuclei) in water and lipid. At the atomic level, since the proton is a charged particle which spins around an internal axis of rotation with a given value of angular momentum (P), it also has a magnetic moment (μ), and therefore can be thought of as a very small bar magnet with a north and south pole, as shown in Figure 5.2. The phenomenon of quantization is familiar from basic physics and chemistry, and means that certain physical parameters can take on only discrete values, rather than having a continuous range. Examples include electric charge, the energy of a photon, and quantum numbers of electrons. Relevant to MRI, the magnitude of the angular momentum of the proton is quantized and has a single, fixed value. The magnitude of the proton's magnetic moment is proportional to the magnitude of the angular momentum:

$$|\vec{\mu}| = \gamma |\vec{P}|, \tag{5.1}$$

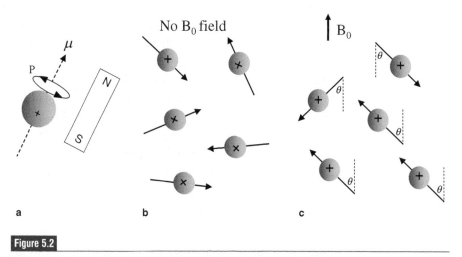

Figure 5.2

(a) The internal rotation of a proton creates a magnetic moment, and so the proton acts as a magnet with north and south pole. (b) In the absence of a strong magnetic field, the orientations of the magnetic moments are completely random. (c) When there is a strong magnetic field present the magnetic moments must align at an angle $\theta = \pm54.7°$ with respect to the direction of B_0.

where γ is a constant called the gyromagnetic ratio, and has a value of 267.54 MHz/Tesla for protons. As a result, the magnitude of the magnetic moment has a single, fixed value. Outside the MRI magnet, as shown in Figure 5.2 the magnitude of the magnetic moment of every proton in our bodies is fixed, but the orientation is completely random. Therefore, the net magnetization, i.e. the sum of all the individual magnetic moments in our bodies, is zero (ignoring the very small effects from the earth's magnetic field).

The situation changes when the patient is slid into the magnet for an MRI scan. From quantum mechanics, the component of the magnetic moment in the direction of B_0 can have only two discrete values, which results in the magnetic moments being aligned at an angle of 54.7° with respect to the direction B_0, aligned either in the same direction or in the opposite direction, as shown in Figure 5.2(c). The former configuration is termed as the parallel, and the latter as the anti-parallel configuration: note however that the terms parallel and anti-parallel only refer to the z-component of μ, and that μ is actually aligned at an angle with respect to B_0.

The relative number of protons in the parallel and anti-parallel configurations depends upon the value of B_0. Protons in the parallel configuration are in the more energy 'favourable' state, compared to the anti-parallel configuration. The energy difference (ΔE) between the two states is shown in Figure 5.3 and given by:

$$\Delta E = \frac{\gamma h B_0}{2\pi}, \tag{5.2}$$

where h is Plank's constant (6.63×10^{-34} J s). To calculate the relative number of protons in each of the two configurations the Boltzmann equation can be used:

$$\frac{N_{anti\text{-}parallel}}{N_{parallel}} = \exp - \left[\frac{\Delta E}{kT}\right] = \exp - \left[\frac{\gamma h B_0}{2\pi kT}\right]. \tag{5.3}$$

where k is Boltzmann's constant with a value of 1.38×10^{-23} J/K, and T is the temperature measured in Kelvin. Since the value of the exponent is very small, a first order approximation, $e^{-x} \approx 1 - x$, can be made:

$$\frac{N_{anti\text{-}parallel}}{N_{parallel}} = 1 - \left[\frac{\gamma h B_0}{2\pi kT}\right]. \tag{5.4}$$

The MRI signal depends upon the difference in populations between the two energy levels:

$$N_{parallel} - N_{anti\text{-}parallel} = N_{total} \frac{\gamma h B_0}{4\pi kT}, \tag{5.5}$$

where N_{total} is the total number of protons. It is important to note that MRI can detect only the *difference* $N_{parallel} - N_{anti\text{-}parallel}$, and not the total number of protons.

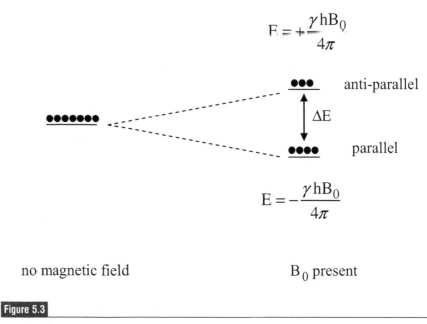

$$E = +\frac{\gamma hB_0}{4\pi}$$

anti-parallel

ΔE

parallel

$$E = -\frac{\gamma hB_0}{4\pi}$$

no magnetic field B_0 present

Figure 5.3

Proton configurations. (left) In the absence of a strong magnetic field, the energies of all the random orientations of the magnetic moments are the same. (right) When a strong magnetic field is applied, the single energy level splits into two levels, one corresponding to the magnetic moments being in the parallel state, and the other the anti-parallel state. The energy difference between the two levels depends upon the value of B_0. There are slightly more protons (shown as filled circles) in the parallel ground energy state than in the higher energy anti-parallel state.

Example 5.1   Assuming a value of room temperature of 25 °C, what is the value of $N_{parallel}$-$N_{anti\text{-}parallel}$ for the head at 3 Tesla, and what percentage of N_{total} does this represent? Assume that the head is spherical with diameter 20 cm and consists entirely of water.

Solution   The volume of the head is given by $4/3\ \pi r^3 = 4189$ cm^3. Since we assume that the head is entirely water, with density 1 g/cm^3, the mass of protons in the head is 4189 g. The atomic mass of water is 18, which means that there are 4189/18 = 232.7 moles of water in the head. Using Avogadro's number, each mole has 6.02×10^{23} protons and so in the head there are 1.4×10^{26} protons. This is the value of N_{total} in Equation (5.5). Now, plugging the values of the constants into Equation (5.5):

$$N_{parallel} - N_{anti\text{-}parallel} = 1.4 \times 10^{26}\frac{267.54 \times 10^6 (\text{HzT}^{-1})6.63 \times 10^{-34}(\text{Js})3(\text{T})}{4\pi \times 1.38 \times 10^{-34}(\text{JK}^{-1})298(\text{K})}.$$

$$= 1.44 \times 10^{21}$$

The MRI signal, as a percentage of the total number of protons is given by:

$$\frac{N_{parallel} - N_{anti\text{-}parallel}}{N_{total}} = 1 \times 10^{-5}.$$

In other words, out of every 1 million protons, only the small difference of 10 protons between the parallel and anti-parallel energy states can be measured.

5.2.2 Classical precession

Having determined that the proton magnetic moments are all aligned at an angle of 54.7° with respect to the direction of B_0, the motion of these magnetic moments can most easily be described using classical mechanics. The B_0 field attempts to align the proton magnetic moment with itself, and this action creates a torque, C, given by the cross product of the two magnetic fields:

$$\overrightarrow{C} = \overrightarrow{\mu} \times \overrightarrow{B_0} = i_N |\mu||B_0|\sin\theta, \qquad (5.6)$$

where i_N is a unit vector normal to both $\overrightarrow{\mu}$ and $\overrightarrow{B_0}$. The direction of the torque, shown in Figure 5.4, is tangential to the direction of $\overrightarrow{\mu}$ and so causes the proton to 'precess' around the axis of the magnetic field, while keeping a constant angle of 54.7° between $\overrightarrow{\mu}$ and $\overrightarrow{B_0}$. An everyday analogue of this motion is a spinning top or gyroscope, where gravity is the external force acting in the vertical direction. Provided that the top is spinning around its internal axis, it precesses by sweeping around a conical trajectory at a constant angle.

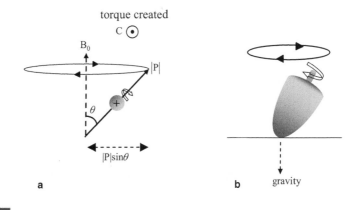

Figure 5.4

A proton in a magnetic field. (a) Using classical mechanics, the torque C acting on the magnetic moment, spinning about an internal axis, causes it to precess about the vertical axis, B_0. (b) A familiar analogy is that of a spinning top: in this case the vertical force is gravity.

To calculate how fast a proton precesses, we use the fact that the torque is defined as the time rate of change of the proton's angular momentum:

$$\vec{C} = \frac{d\vec{P}}{dt} = \vec{\mu} \times \vec{B_0}. \tag{5.7}$$

From Figure 5.4, the magnitude of the component of the angular momentum which precesses in the plane perpendicular to B_0 is given by $\left|\vec{P}\right| \sin\theta$. In a short time dt, μ precesses through an angle $d\varphi$ resulting in a change $d\vec{P}$ in the angular momentum. Simple trigonometry gives the relationship that:

$$\sin(d\varphi) = \frac{d\vec{P}}{\left|\vec{P}\right|\sin\theta} = \frac{\vec{C}dt}{\left|\vec{P}\right|\sin\theta}. \tag{5.8}$$

If $d\varphi$ is small then we can make the approximation that $\sin(d\varphi) = d\varphi$. The angular precession frequency, ω, is given by $d\varphi/dt$ and so has a value:

$$\omega = \frac{d\varphi}{dt} = \frac{\vec{C}}{\left|\vec{P}\right|\sin\theta} = \frac{\vec{\mu} \times \vec{B_0}}{\left|\vec{P}\right|\sin\theta} = \frac{\gamma\vec{P} \times \vec{B_0}}{\left|\vec{P}\right|\sin\theta} = \frac{\gamma\left|\vec{P}\right|\left|\vec{B_0}\right|\sin\theta}{\left|\vec{P}\right|\sin\theta} = \gamma B_0.$$

$$\tag{5.9}$$

The effect of placing a proton in a magnetic field, therefore, is to cause it to precess around B_0 at a frequency directly proportional to the strength of the magnetic field. This frequency, termed ω_0, is termed the Larmor frequency after the renowned Irish physicist Joseph Larmor.

Example 5.2   What are the Larmor frequencies, expressed in MHz, for B_0 fields of 1.5 Tesla, 3 Tesla and 7 Tesla?

Solution   For 1.5 Tesla, the frequency is given by:

$$f = \frac{\omega}{2\pi} = \frac{\gamma B_0}{2\pi} = \frac{267.54 \times 10^6 (HzT^{-1})1.5(T)}{2\pi} = 63.9 \text{ MHz}.$$

Simple multiplication gives frequencies (rounded to one significant figure) of 127.7 and 298.1 MHz for 3 Tesla and 7 Tesla, respectively.

By combining the results of the quantum mechanical and classical analysis we can represent the net magnetization from the entire patient in a simple vector form. Figure 5.5 shows on the left a representation of several proton magnetic moments,

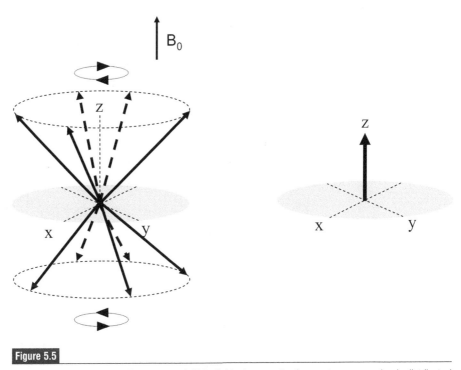

Figure 5.5

Magnetization represented by vectors. (left) Individual magnetization vectors are randomly distributed around a cone which subtends an angle of 54.7° with respect to the B_0 (z) axis. The vector sum of all of the individual magnetization vectors (right) is simply a static component in the direction of B_0.

each aligned at 54.7° to B_0, each precessing at a frequency ω_0, with slightly more protons in the parallel than anti-parallel state. The total magnetization can be calculated by a simple vector sum of the individual components, and is shown on the right of Figure 5.5. It can be seen that the net magnetization has only a z-component, since the vector sum of the components on the x- and y-axes is zero.

The net magnetization of the sample is defined as M_0:

$$M_0 = \sum_{n=1}^{N_{total}} \mu_{z,n} = \frac{\gamma h}{4\pi} \left(N_{parallel} - N_{anti\text{-}parallel} \right) = \frac{\gamma^2 h^2 B_0 N_{total}}{16\pi^2 kT}. \qquad (5.10)$$

5.3 Effects of a radiofrequency pulse on magnetization

The energy levels for protons in a magnetic field, shown in Figure 5.3, are analogous to energy levels in semiconductors and also the vibrational and rotational energy levels used in infrared spectroscopy. As with all such multi-level systems, to obtain an MR signal, energy must be supplied with a specific value ΔE, given by Equation (5.2), to stimulate transitions between the energy levels. The energy is supplied as an electromagnetic (EM), usually referred to as a radiofrequency (RF) field, the frequency (f) of which can be calculated from De Broglie's relationship, ΔE–hf.

$$hf = \Delta E = \frac{\gamma h B_0}{2\pi}$$

$$\Rightarrow f = \frac{\gamma B_0}{2\pi} \text{ or } \omega = \gamma B_0 \tag{5.11}$$

By comparing Equations (5.11) and (5.9) it can be seen that the frequency of the RF field is identical to the precession frequency.

5.3.1 Creation of transverse magnetization

In MRI, energy is applied as a short RF pulse, with the direction of the magnetic component of the RF field oriented at 90° to the direction of B_0, as shown in Figure 5.6. Applying the same classical analysis as for proton precession, the magnetic component of the RF pulse, termed the B_1 field, produces a torque which causes the net magnetization to rotate towards the xy-plane as shown in Figure 5.6. Note that if the B_1 field is applied along the x-axis, the magnetic moment vector is rotated towards the y-axis (see Exercise 5.2).

The 'tip angle' (α) is defined as the angle through which the net magnetization is rotated. This angle is proportional to both the strength of the applied RF field (measured in Tesla) and the time, τ_{B1}, for which it is applied:

$$\alpha = \gamma B_1 \tau_{B1}. \tag{5.12}$$

A tip angle of 90°, termed a 90° pulse, results in the maximum value of the M_y component of magnetization, whereas one of 180° produces no M_y magnetization but rotates the net magnetization M_0 from the +z to the − z axis.

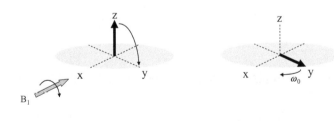

Figure 5.6

(left) Application of an RF pulse about the x-axis rotates the magnetization from the z-direction towards the y-axis. If the RF pulse strength and duration are chosen to produce a 90° pulse, then the magnetization lies directly along the y-axis. When the RF pulse is switched off (right), the magnetization precesses around the z-axis at the Larmor frequency ω_0.

Example 5.3 In MRI a typical B_1 field is 30 microTesla, calculate how long this B_1 field must be applied to produce a 90° pulse.

Solution The problem is most easily solved by using units of radians for the tip angle, where an angle of $\pi/2$ radians is equivalent to 90°. Using Equation (5.12):

$$\tau_{B1} = \frac{\alpha}{\gamma B_1} = \frac{\pi/2}{267.54 \times 10^6 (HzT^{-1})30 \times 10^{-6}(T)} = 1.96 \times 10^{-4}s.$$

5.4 Faraday induction: the basis of MR signal detection

In the most simple case, the MR detector consists of a pair of conductive loops (of copper wire for example) placed close to the patient at an angle of 90° with respect to each other. Faraday's law of induction states that a voltage (V) is induced in each of these loops with a value proportional to the time rate of change of the magnetic flux $d\varphi$:

$$V \propto -\frac{d\varphi}{dt}. \tag{5.13}$$

Figure 5.7 shows the situation a short time after a 90° pulse has been applied about the x-axis: in this case the respective voltages induced in the two coils are given by:

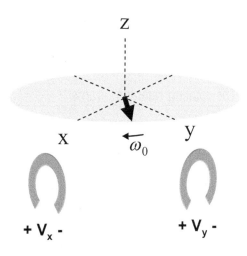

Figure 5.7

The MR signal is measured via Faraday induction. Either one or two RF coils can be used, with a voltage being induced across the ends of the conductor loops by the precessing magnetization.

$$V_y \propto M_0 \omega_0 \sin \omega_0 t$$
$$V_x \propto -M_0 \omega_0 \cos \omega_0 t$$

(5.14)

It is important to note that the requirement for a *time-varying* magnetic flux to induce an MR signal is the reason why only magnetization precessing in the xy-plane gives rise to an MR signal. Any z-component of magnetization does not precess and therefore does not induce a voltage.

5.4.1 MR signal intensity

The size of the MR signal is determined by three different factors. First, the signal is proportional to the number of protons in the object, from Equation (5.5). In terms of MRI, as will be seen later, this corresponds to the number of protons in each voxel of the image. The other two factors depend upon the value of the B_0 field. From Equation (5.10), the value of M_0 is proportional to B_0: therefore a 3 Tesla MRI system has twice the M_0 of a 1.5 Tesla system. Also, from Equation (5.14), the induced voltage is proportional to the precession frequency, which in turn is proportional to B_0. Overall, therefore, the MR signal is proportional to the square of the B_0 field, one of the reasons why there is such a strong drive towards higher field MRI systems. Of course, in terms of the overall SNR, the dependence of the noise on the strength of the B_0 field must also be considered: this is covered in detail in Section 5.20.1. Overall, the image SNR is proportional to the 3/2 power of the value of the B_0 field.

5.4.2 The rotating reference frame

The x and y components of transverse magnetization (M_x and M_y) precess around B_0 at a very high frequency, ~128 MHz for a 3 Tesla magnet. In terms of visualizing this motion the concept of a 'rotating reference frame' (x',y',z) is extremely useful, see Figure 5.8. In this frame the x'y' plane rotates around the z-axis at the Larmor frequency. Therefore, protons precessing at the Larmor frequency appear static in the rotating reference frame. Although the transformation is trivial when considering protons precessing at a single frequency, during imaging sequences protons precess at different frequencies depending upon their spatial location, and then the rotating reference frame becomes essential for analysis. It should be emphasized that the rotating reference frame is only a convenient visualization *model*: in reality all protons precess around B_0.

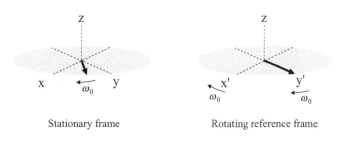

Stationary frame   Rotating reference frame

Relationship between the stationary frame (left) and the rotating frame (right). In the stationary frame the magnetization precesses in the transverse plane around the z-axis at an angular frequency of ω_0 radians/sec. In the rotating reference frame it is the axes themselves (x′,y′) that rotate around the z-axis at ω_0 radians/sec, and therefore the magnetization appears stationary.

5.5 T_1 and T_2 relaxation times

As seen in Section 5.2, the equilibrium magnetization state corresponds to a z-component, M_z, equal to M_0 and transverse components, M_x and M_y, equal to zero. Application of an RF pulse creates a non-equilibrium state by adding energy to the system. After the pulse has been switched off, the system must relax back to thermal equilibrium. The phenomenon of relaxation is familiar from many engineering applications: for example, the application of an impulse voltage pulse to an RC electrical circuit produces time-varying voltages across the lumped elements, the values of which return in time to their values prior to the pulse being applied, this process being characterized by certain time-constants. Figure 5.9 shows what happens to the magnetization after application of a 90° pulse around the x axis.

It is important to note that there are two relaxation times which govern the return to equilibrium of the z-component, and the x- and y-components, respectively. These are referred to as T_1-relaxation (which affects only z-magnetization) and T_2-relaxation (which affects only x- and y-magnetization). These are also called spin-lattice (T_1) and spin-spin (T_2) relaxation. MR relaxation is described mathematically by relatively simple first order differential equations known as the Bloch equations [1]. Solutions of these equations give the following relationships: after an RF pulse of arbitrary tip angle α, the value of M_z at a time t is given by:

$$M_z(t) = M_0 \cos \alpha + (M_0 - M_0 \cos \alpha)\left(1 - e^{-\frac{t}{T_1}}\right). \tag{5.15}$$

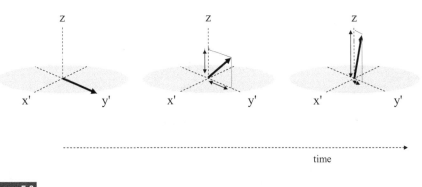

Figure 5.9

(left) Magnetization vector after a 90° RF pulse about the x-axis. (centre) T_1 and T_2 relaxation of the magnetization a certain time after the pulse has been applied results in an increased M_z component and reduced M_y component, respectively. (right) After a further time, the M_z and M_y components have almost returned to their equilibrium values of M_0 and zero, respectively.

For example, after a 90° pulse the value of M_z is given by:

$$M_z(t) = M_0 \left(1 - e^{-\frac{t}{T_1}} \right). \tag{5.16}$$

Different tissues have different values of T_1, and diseased tissues often have substantially altered T_1 relaxation time compared to healthy tissue, and these differences form one basis for introducing contrast into the MR image. Values of tissue T_1 values for 1.5 and 3 Tesla are shown in Table 5.1. It can be seen that the values of T_1 depend not only upon tissue type but also the magnetic field strength, a topic covered more fully in Section 5.13.

Figure 5.10 shows the time dependence of the M_z magnetization after a 90° pulse for two tissues with different T_1 values.

The second relaxation time, T_2, governs the return of the M_x and M_y components of magnetization to their thermal equilibrium values of zero. If an RF pulse of arbitrary tip angle α is applied along the x-axis, the value of M_y at time t after the RF pulse is given by:

$$M_y(t) = M_0 \sin \alpha \, \exp - \left(\frac{t}{T_2} \right). \tag{5.17}$$

As is the case for T_1 relaxation times, different tissues in the body have different values of T_2, and these can also be used to differentiate between healthy and diseased tissues in clinical images. Similarly to T_1, the values of T_2 also depend on B_0, and Table 5.1 shows typical values at 1.5 and 3 Tesla. It should be noted that there is no direct correlation between the T_1 and T_2 values, a long T_1 does not necessarily mean a long T_2. The only thing that is universally true, detailed further in Section 5.13, is that T_1 is always greater than T_2.

Table 5.1: Tissue relaxation times (ms) at 1.5 and 3 Tesla

Tissue	T_1 (1.5 T)	T_1 (3 T)	T_2 (1.5 T)	T_2 (3 T)
Brain (white matter)	790	1100	90	60
Brain (grey matter)	920	1600	100	80
Liver	500	800	50	40
Skeletal muscle	870	1420	60	30
Lipid (subcutaneous)	290	360	160	130
Cartilage	1060	1240	42	37

short TR

all long TE

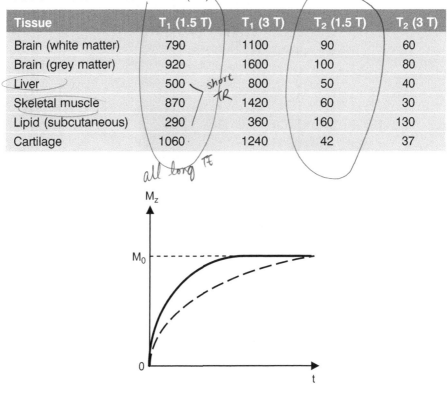

Figure 5.10

The recovery of M_z magnetization as a function of time after a 90° pulse for a tissue with short T_1 relaxation time (solid line) and long T_1 relaxation time (dashed line). When $t = 5*T_1$, $M_z \sim 99\%$ M_0, which is assumed to be full recovery.

The mechanism that gives rise to T_2 relaxation is shown in Figure 5.11. Although it has been assumed that all protons precess at exactly the same frequency, in practice molecular dynamics means that there is a small spread in the precessional frequencies. In the rotating reference frame one can visualize this as the vectors spreading out in time. The phase (φ) of the vector is defined as the angle of the vector with respect to the y′ axis. As the vectors spread out, they accumulate different values of φ, and lose 'phase coherence'. The vector sum of all the individual magnetic moments decreases exponentially, and when the vectors are randomly located around the transverse plane, the MR signal is zero and therefore the M_x and M_y components have returned to equilibrium.

In practice there is an important additional factor which leads to relaxation of M_x and M_y back to zero. This arises due to spatial inhomogeneities in the B_0 field within the patient. There are two sources for these variations. The first is the fact

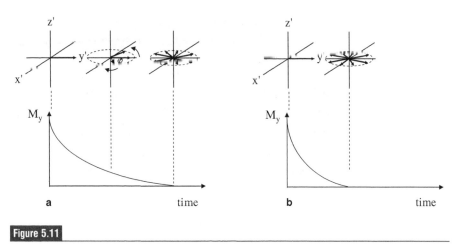

Figure 5.11

The time-dependence of the M_y component of magnetization for (a) a tissue with relatively long T_2^* and (b) one with a shorter T_2^*. The decrease in signal occurs due to the loss of phase coherence of the protons, i.e. protons precess at slightly different frequencies, thus acquiring different phases and reducing the net magnetization along the y-axis. The faster the dephasing process the shorter the T_2^* relaxation time.

that it is not possible to design a magnet which produces a perfectly uniform B_0 field over the entire imaging volume. MR magnets are designed to produce as large a volume of as homogenous a field as possible, as covered in Section 5.14.1, but there are manufacturing and physical limits to the homogeneity that can be achieved. The second source arises from local variations in magnetic field due to the different magnetic susceptibilities of different parts of the body. For example, close to any surgical implant (even if it is constructed from an MRI compatible material such as titanium) the material properties alter the effective B_0 field significantly. This also occurs, albeit to a lesser extent, at interfaces between tissues with very different properties, for example near air cavities in the head (air is paramagnetic due to its oxygen content). If there are large local variations in the B_0 field, then from Equation (5.9) there are large variations in the proton precession frequencies, which will cause much more rapid dephasing of the magnetization than pure T_2 relaxation. The effects of local B_0 field inhomogeneity are characterized by a relaxation time T_2^+. The combined relaxation time is designated by T_2^*, the value of which is given by:

$$\frac{1}{T_2^*} = \frac{1}{T_2^+} + \frac{1}{T_2}.$$

(5.18)

In MRI, T_2^* values can vary from less than a millisecond close to a metallic implant, to tens of milliseconds near air/tissue interfaces, to hundreds of milliseconds for very homogeneous tissue in the brain.

5.6 Signals from lipid

The assumption so far has been that all protons in the body resonate very close to the same frequency, and this is true for water protons within tissue, However, protons in lipid resonate at a significantly different frequency from those in water. The largest number of protons in lipid are present as $-CH_2-$ groups in long-chain fatty acids. The reason why the resonant frequencies of protons in lipid are different from those in water is that the strength of the magnetic field experienced by a proton depends not only upon the B_0 field strength, but also is affected by the geometry of the electron configuration which surrounds the proton. Analogous to a proton, an electron is a spinning, charged particle and has an electronic magnetic moment which produces a small magnetic field opposite in polarity (since it is negatively charged) to the main magnetic field, B_0. This reduces the effective magnetic field, B_{eff}, experienced by the proton:

$$B_{eff} = B_0(1 - \sigma),\tag{5.19}$$

where σ is called the shielding constant, and is related to the electronic environment surrounding the nucleus. The resonant frequency of the proton is given by:

$$\omega = \gamma B_{eff} = \gamma B_0(1 - \sigma).\tag{5.20}$$

As shown in Figure 5.12, lipid (-CH_2-) and water (H_2O) have different electron distributions around the protons, due primarily to the different electronegativities of the oxygen and carbon atoms, and so the protons in the two species resonate at different frequencies. Since oxygen is much more electronegative than carbon, electrons are pulled away from the protons in water more so than in lipid, and

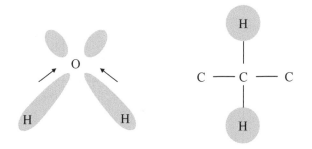

Figure 5.12

The electron density distribution (shaded area) surrounding protons in water and lipid. The strong electronegativity of the oxygen atom in water pulls electrons away from the proton, leaving it unshielded compared to the protons in lipid.

the water protons are less shielded. This means that the value of σ for water is less than that for lipid, and the resonant frequency is higher. At 3 Tesla the difference in resonance frequencies is roughly 2500 rad s^{-1} or 400 Hz.

5.7 The free induction decay

Combining the phenomena of the effects of an RF pulse, MR relaxation, chemical shift, and detection via Faraday induction, the measured MR signal from a human subject is shown in Figure 5.13. This is often referred to as the free induction decay (FID), the name referring to the fact that the signal precesses freely after the RF pulse has been turned off, it is detected via electromagnetic induction, and decays to a zero equilibrium value. If two coils are present then both the M_x and M_y components of magnetization can be detected separately, as shown earlier. It is most convenient to look at the signals in the frequency-domain, rather than time-domain, and this is performed using a Fourier transform of the time-domain signal, as covered in Chapter 1. Figure 5.13 shows the real part of the Fourier transformed MR spectrum. There are two frequencies, as expected, corresponding to protons in lipid (lower frequency) and water (higher frequency). These peaks are not sharp delta functions, but have a Lorenzian lineshape arising from the Fourier transform of the exponentially decaying function. The linewidth of each peak is given by $1/\pi T_2{}^*$.

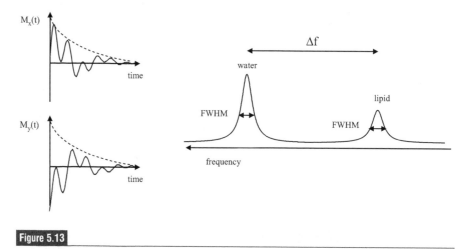

Figure 5.13

(left) x- and y-components of magnetization as a function of time, showing 'beat patterns' which come from the two different resonant frequencies of lipid and water. The real part of the frequency spectrum, shown on the right, shows the two peaks separated by Δf Hz.

5.8 Magnetic resonance imaging

The signal shown in Figure 5.13 contains no spatial information, i.e. there is no way to distinguish between signals coming from protons located at different spatial positions within the body. The concept of making MR an imaging modality originated relatively recently [2] with the realization that if the magnetic field could be made to vary spatially within the subject, this would in turn impose a spatial variation in resonant frequencies that could be exploited to form an image. Such spatial variations have to be varied dynamically. This is performed by incorporating three separate 'gradient coils', described in detail in Section 5.14.2, into the design of an MRI scanner. These gradient coils are designed so that the spatial variation in magnetic field is linear with respect to spatial location, i.e.

$$\frac{\partial B_z}{\partial z} = G_z, \quad \frac{\partial B_z}{\partial x} = G_x, \quad \frac{\partial B_z}{\partial y} = G_y, \tag{5.21}$$

where G represents the gradient measured in T/m. The three separate magnetic field gradients are produced by passing a DC current through separate coils of wire. An example of a coil design which produces a linear gradient in the z-direction is shown in Figure 5.14. The current in each set of gradient coils comes from high-power gradient amplifiers which supply hundreds of amps: the current can be turned on and off very quickly under computer control. The gradient coils are also designed such that there is no additional contribution to the magnetic field at the isocenter ($z = 0$, $y = 0$, $x = 0$) of the gradients, which means that the magnetic field at this position is simply B_0. By convention, the y-axis corresponds to the anterior/posterior direction, and the x-axis to the left/right direction of a patient lying in the magnet. The gradient coils are permanently fixed to the inside of the superconducting magnet, as explained more fully in Section 5.14. Figure 5.14 shows a plot of magnetic field vs. spatial position for a gradient applied along the z-axis.

The magnetic field, B_z, experienced by protons with a common z-coordinate is given by:

$$B_z = B_0 + zG_z. \tag{5.22}$$

From the graph shown in Figure 5.14, at position $z = 0$, $B_z = B_0$; for all positions $z > 0$, $B_z > B_0$, and for positions $z < 0$, $B_z < B_0$. If the direction of the current in the gradient coils were reversed, referred to as applying a negative gradient, then the slope in Figure 5.14 would be negative and for all positions $z > 0$, $B_z < B_0$, and for positions $z < 0$, $B_z > B_0$. The precession frequencies (ω_z) of the protons, as a function of their position in z, are given by:

$$\omega_z = \gamma B_z = \gamma(B_0 + zG_z). \tag{5.23}$$

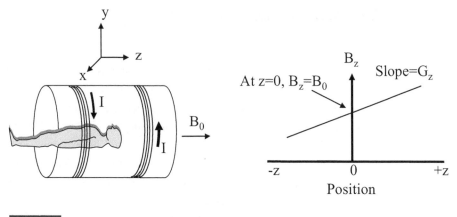

Figure 5.14

(left) A Maxwell-pair gradient coil in which an equal and opposite current is passed through a set of wires which are wound around a cylinder with its major axis in the z-direction. (right) The resulting magnetic field, B_z, is a function of position in z. The slope of the graph is G_z, the z-gradient. Since the currents in the two halves of the gradient coil are equal, the total magnetic field at the centre of the gradient coil is B_0. Applying Fleming's left-hand rule, given the current directions indicated, the total magnetic field is less than B_0 for $z < 0$ and greater than B_0 for $z > 0$.

In the rotating reference frame the precession frequency is:

$$\omega_z = \gamma z G_z, \text{ or } f_z = \frac{\gamma}{2\pi} z G_z. \tag{5.24}$$

Analogous expressions can be obtained for the spatial dependence of the resonant frequencies in the presence of the x- and y-gradients. Typical maximum values of gradient strength on clinical systems are ~40 mT per metre.

Example 5.4 Calculate the resonant frequencies for protons at the top and bottom of the head in a 3 Tesla scanner if a z gradient of 40 mT/m is applied. Assume that the centre of the head is in the centre of the gradient coil, and the head is 25 cm in length. What would be the effect if a negative gradient of -20 mT is applied?

Solution The resonant frequency of protons at the centre of the head is 127.7 MHz, since the additional field from the gradients is zero. For the top of the head, the extra field is given by 0.04 T/m $\times$ 0.125 m = 0.005 T. This corresponds to 0.005 T $\times$ 42.58 MHz/T ~213 kHz. For the bottom of the head the corresponding number is obviously -213 kHz. Therefore, the overall spread is ~426 kHz. If a negative gradient of -20 mT/m is applied, then the spread will be one-half that calculated previously, or 213 kHz. However, protons at the top of the head now resonate at a frequency 106.5 kHz lower than those at the centre of the head, and protons at the bottom of the head resonate 106.5 kHz higher than those at the centre.

5.9 Image acquisition

The process of image formation can be broken down into three separate, independent components, slice selection, phase-encoding and frequency-encoding, covered in the following sections. An overall imaging 'pulse sequence' is shown in Figure 5.15 (a). The transmitter line indicates when an RF pulse is applied, and the length and power of the pulse are adjusted to give the indicated tip angle. For each gradient line, the height of the gradient pulse indicates its strength, and the polarity (positive or negative) indicates which direction current is flowing through the particular gradient coil. The A/D line shows when the receiver is gated on, and how many data points (N_f) are acquired while the frequency encoding gradient is turned on. The entire sequence of RF pulse and three gradients has to be repeated a number of times (N_p typically is between 128 and 512) to build-up a two-dimensional data set, with the arrow next to the phase encoding gradient indicating that different values are used for each repetition of the sequence. Since each of the three components can be treated completely independently, gradient events in practice are overlapped to reduce the overall time of the imaging sequence, as shown in Figure 5.15 (b).

5.9.1 Slice selection

The first part of planning an MRI scanning session is to decide in which orientation the slice should be acquired. Unlike in CT, in which axial sections are always

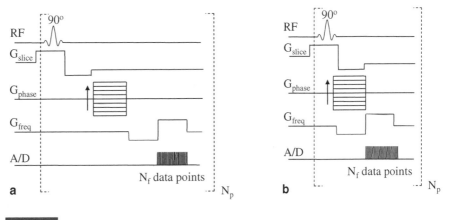

Figure 5.15

Pulse sequence diagrams for imaging sequences. An RF pulse is applied, various gradients are turned on and off, and the analogue-to-digital (A/D) converter is gated on to acquire data. (a) Individual steps in image formation can be considered independently in terms of slice selection (RF and G_{slice}), phase encoding (G_{phase}) and frequency encoding (G_{freq} and the A/D on). (b) In practice, the gradients are applied simultaneously where appropriate in order to minimize the time between RF excitation and signal acquisition.

acquired, MRI can acquire the image in any given orientation. For example, coronal, axial or sagittal images, corresponding to slice-selection in the y-, z, or x directions, respectively, can be chosen, as shown in Figure 5.16. In practice, different clinical imaging protocols of various parts of the body call for different image orientations.

Slice selection uses a frequency-selective RF pulse applied simultaneously with one of the magnetic field gradients (G_x, G_y or G_z), denoted by G_{slice}. The selective RF pulse is applied at a specific frequency ω_s, with an excitation bandwidth of $\pm\Delta\omega_s$. This is analogous to a radio station transmitter, which transmits energy at a certain frequency over a limited bandwidth. Protons which have a precession frequency within the bandwidth (between $\omega_s + \Delta\omega_s$ and $\omega_s - \Delta\omega_s$) are rotated into the transverse plane by the RF pulse, but protons with precession frequencies outside the bandwidth are not affected. Figure 5.17 shows the orientation of the protons after a 90° pulse, assuming that an axial slice was chosen.

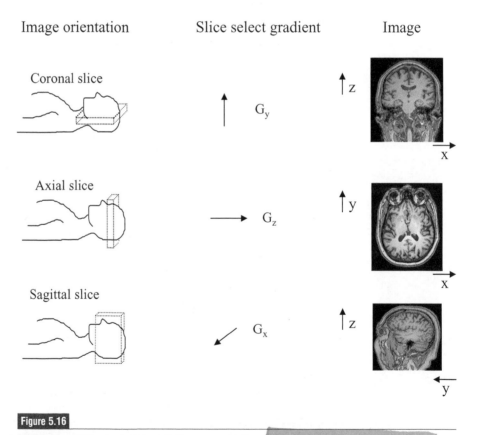

Image orientation	Slice select gradient	Image
Coronal slice	G_y	
Axial slice	G_z	
Sagittal slice	G_x	

Figure 5.16

Showing the different orientations for image acquisition. Coronal (top), axial (middle) or sagittal (bottom) slices can be produced by turning on the y, z, or x gradients, respectively, while the RF pulse is being applied.

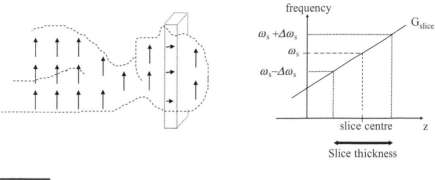

Figure 5.17

(left) The effects of a 90° RF pulse applied simultaneously with the z-gradient. Only protons within the axial slice are tipped by 90° into the transverse plane, and so give a measureable MR signal. Protons outside the chosen slice have their net magnetization remain in the z-direction. (right) Showing the gradient strength (the slope of the graph) as a function of position in z.

The slice thickness (T) is given by:

$$T = \frac{2\Delta\omega_s}{\gamma G_{slice}}. \tag{5.25}$$

The slice can therefore be made thinner either by increasing the strength of G_{slice} (up to its maximum value) or decreasing the frequency bandwidth of the RF pulse. The ideal frequency excitation profile of the RF pulse is a rectangular shape, in which case an equal tip angle is applied to all the protons within the slice, and zero tip angle to protons outside the slice. Using the Fourier transform properties in Section 1.9.1, a sinc or similarly shaped RF pulse, typically with a length of a few ms, is used. The slice position can be moved to different parts of the patient by changing the value of ω_s of the RF pulse.

Example 5.5   If the maximum gradient strength is 40 mT/m, calculate the bandwidth of the RF pulse necessary to give a 1 mm slice thickness. If the slice thickness is decreased to 0.5 mm, is the required RF pulse shorter or longer than for a 1 mm slice thickness?

Solution   Using Equation (5.23):

$$1 \times 10^{-3}(\text{m}) = \frac{2\Delta\omega_s}{267.54 \times 10^6\,(\text{HzT}^{-1})0.04\,(\text{Tm}^{-1})}.$$

Solving gives a bandwidth $2\Delta\omega_s$ of 10 070 rads^{-1} or 1700 Hz.
From the properties of the Fourier transform, a longer RF pulse results in a narrower frequency spectrum, and therefore the thinner slice requires an RF pulse of double the length for a given value of G_{slice}.

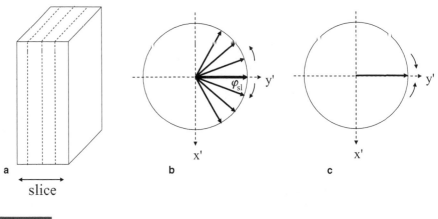

Figure 5.18

(a) Since the slice has a finite thickness, protons at different z-positions within the slice precess at different frequencies during the RF pulse. (b) At the end of the RF pulse protons at each z-position have acquired a phase φ_{sl} given by Equation (5.26), and the net magnetization vector is reduced significantly due to the lack of phase coherence. (c) Application of a negative rephasing slice gradient of the appropriate duration and strength refocuses all the magnetization to give the maximum net magnetization.

Analyzing the motion of the protons within the slice more closely, due to the fact that the RF pulse is relatively long (typically 1 millisecond or longer), protons at different z-positions within the slice precess around B_0 during the pulse, and therefore accumulate different phases (φ_{slice}), as shown in Figure 5.18:

$$\varphi_{\mathrm{slice}}(z) = \gamma G_z z \frac{\tau}{2}, \tag{5.26}$$

where τ is the duration of the RF pulse. The net magnetization, given by the vector sum of all the individual vectors, is reduced compared to its value if the RF pulse were very short. Fortunately, there is a simple way to 'reverse' this dephasing of the magnetization. A negative rephasing gradient (G_{slice}^{ref}) is applied for a time τ^{ref}. Assuming that the gradient waveforms are perfectly rectangular, complete refocusing occurs when:

$$G_{\mathrm{slice}}^{\mathrm{ref}} \tau^{\mathrm{ref}} = \frac{\tau}{2} G_z. \tag{5.27}$$

5.9.2 Phase encoding

Continuing with the example of an axial slice, in which the slice select gradient was applied in the z-direction, the x and y directions are now encoded via the phase and frequency of the MR signal [3,4]. For a simple imaging sequence it is not important which dimension is encoded by the phase and which by the frequency. As shown in Figure 5.15, a phase encoding gradient (G_{phase}) is turned on for a period τ_{pe} and then switched off. If G_{phase} corresponds to the y-dimension, during the interval τ_{pe} the protons precess at a frequency $\omega_y = \gamma G_y y$. The net effect is to introduce a spatially dependent phase shift, $\varphi_{pe}(G_y, \tau_{pe})$, with a value given by:

$$\varphi_{pe}\left(G_y, \tau_{pe}\right) = \omega_y \tau_{pe} = \gamma G_y y \tau_{pe}. \tag{5.28}$$

This is shown in Figure 5.19, for five protons at positions y = 0, +1, +2, +3, and +4 cm with respect to the centre of the gradient coil. The value of the first phase encoding gradient, G_{pe1}, corresponds to the maximum negative gradient step, as shown in Figure 5.15. This induces different phase shifts, where $\varphi_2 = 2\varphi_1$, $\varphi_3 = 3\varphi_1$, and $\varphi_4 = 4\varphi_1$, as shown in Figure 5.19. The second value of the phase encoding gradient, G_{pe2}, corresponds to a value slightly less negative than G_{pe1}, with the difference given by ΔG_{pe}. The phase shifts at each y-position are therefore slightly less than for G_{pe1}.

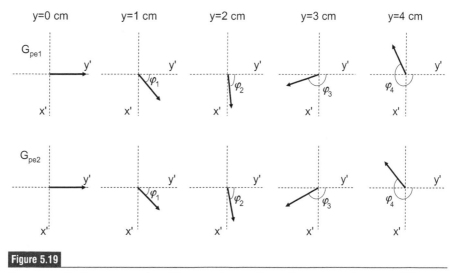

Figure 5.19

Phase encoding for protons at four different vertical positions with respect to the centre of the y-gradient. In the upper panel, a gradient G_{pe1} is applied. Protons at the very centre of the y-gradient experience no additional magnetic field and so accumulate no phase in the rotating reference frame. The larger the offset in the y-dimension, the larger the phase shift accumulated. In the lower panel, the next value of the phase encoding gradient is applied, with G_{pe2} being slightly less negative than G_{pe1}. Again, protons at y=0 accumulate no phase, and protons at different y-positions accumulate phases slightly lower in value than when G_{pe1} was applied. Typically between 128 and 512 different values of G_{pe} are used to acquire the full image.

5.9.3 Frequency encoding

The x-dimension is encoded by applying a frequency-encoding gradient (G_{freq}) while the receiver is gated on and data are being acquired. During this time t, protons precess at a frequency given by $\omega_x = \gamma G_x x$ determined only by their x-location. A total of N_f data points are acquired while the receiver is on.

Overall, this means that for each phase encoding step each voxel in the image is characterized by a specific phase which depends upon its position in y, and specific frequency which depends upon its position in x, as shown in Figure 5.20.

To form, for example, a 256×256 image, $N_f = 256$ and the sequence must be repeated 256 times, each time with a different value of the phase encoding gradient, ranging from its maximum negative to maximum positive value in equal increments of ΔG_{pe}. In order for sufficient T_1 relaxation to occur so that a significant fraction of M_z magnetization recovers between successive RF excitations, there is a delay between successive RF pulses, called the TR (time of repetition)

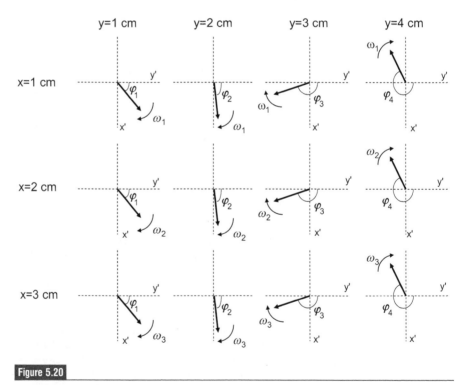

Figure 5.20

Combined effect of phase and frequency encoding gradients. The phases accumulated by protons at a given y-position are identical to those shown in Figure 5.19. During data acquisition the frequencies at which the protons precess are linearly dependent upon their position in the x-dimension. In this case $\omega_2 = 2\omega_1$ and $\omega_3 = 3\omega_1$.

time. Overall, the total data acquisition time is therefore given by the TR multiplied by the number of phase encoding steps applied, $TR*N_{pe}$.

5.10   The k-space formalism and image reconstruction

To understand how the acquired data are transformed into an image, it is instructive to express the ($N_f \times N_{pe}$) signals mathematically as

$$s(G_y, \tau_{pe}, G_x, t) \propto \int_{slice} \int_{slice} \rho(x, y) e^{-j\gamma G_y y \tau_{pe}} e^{-j\gamma G_x x t} dxdy. \tag{5.29}$$

One can treat the slice, phase and frequency encoding terms independently. The double integral over the slice represents the fact that signal comes only from protons within the slice, and that there is no signal from protons outside this slice. The factor $\rho(x,y)$ is the number of protons at each position (x,y) within this slice, and is called the proton density. This can be related to the term N_{total} in Equation (5.10): the signal intensity is directly proportional to the number of protons in each voxel. The second term in the integral represents the phase term ($\varphi_y = \gamma G_y y \tau_{pe}$) from the phase encoding gradient. The third term in the equation represents the spatially dependent resonance frequency ($\omega_x = \gamma G_x x$).

A very useful model is the 'k-space' formalism developed by Ljunggren [5]. Two variables, k_x and k_y, are defined as:

$$k_x = \frac{\gamma}{2\pi} G_x t, \ k_y = \frac{\gamma}{2\pi} G_y \tau_{pe}. \tag{5.30}$$

The k values are spatial frequencies, as covered in Chapter 1. Equation (5.29) can now be expressed in terms of these two variables:

$$S(k_x, k_y) \propto \int_{slice} \int_{slice} \rho(x, y) e^{-j2\pi k_x x} e^{-j2\pi k_y y} dxdy. \tag{5.31}$$

The acquired data can therefore be represented as a two-dimensional data set in k_x,k_y-space. Consider the N_f data points collected when the maximum negative value of the phase-encoding gradient, G_y, is applied. From Equation (5.30) the value of k_y for all N_f data points corresponds to its maximum negative value. As shown in Figure 5.15, a negative gradient , is applied in the x-direction before data acquisition. Denoting the strength of this gradient by $G_{dephase}$ and the time for which it is applied by $\tau_{dephase}$, then the values are chosen are chosen such that:

$$G_{dephase}\tau_{dephase} = \frac{T_{acq}}{2} G_{freq}. \tag{5.32}$$

This means that the dephasing gradient is exactly cancelled out at the centre of the acquisition time (T_{acq}). The first data point acquired when the frequency-encoding gradient is switched on corresponds to a negative value of k_x, the second data point to a slightly more positive value of k_x and so forth. After the first $N_f/2$ data points have been acquired k_x reaches a value of 0, and then becomes positive for the remaining $N_f/2$ data points. Therefore, the N_f data points correspond to one 'line' in k-space, shown as line 1 in Figure 5.21. The second line in k-space corresponds to the next value of the phase-encoding gradient, and so is displaced to a more positive value of k_y. In this way, the full two-dimensional k-space matrix is acquired, as shown in Figure 5.21.

How is the image formed from the acquired k-space data? In Section 1.9.1 the inverse Fourier transform of a function $S(k_x,k_y)$ was given by:

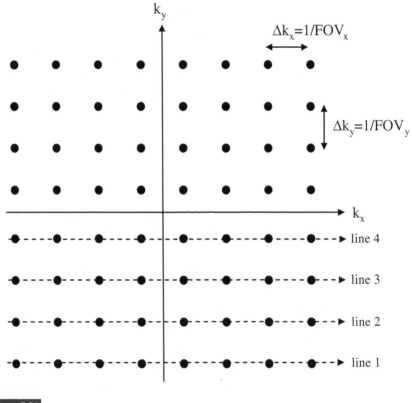

Figure 5.21

k-space: data acquisition occurs line-by-line, with the first line acquired corresponding to the maximum negative value of the phase encoding gradient. The values of Δk_x and Δk_y between successive data points are equal to the inverse of the respective fields-of-view of the image (see Exercise 5.15).

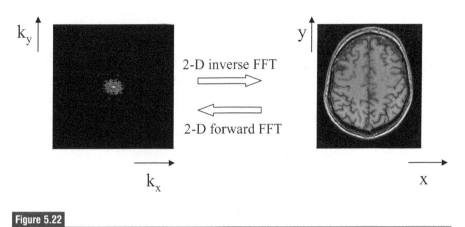

k_y 2-D inverse FFT y

2-D forward FFT

k_x x

Figure 5.22

The mathematical relationship between the acquired k-space data on the left and the image on the right is a two-dimensional Fourier-transform. Although both the k-space data and image data are complex with real and imaginary components, they are both typically illustrated in magnitude mode.

$$\rho(x, y) = \int\limits_{-\infty}^{\infty} \int\limits_{-\infty}^{\infty} S\left(k_x, k_y\right) e^{+j2\pi\left(k_x x + k_y y\right)} dk_x dk_y. \qquad (5.33)$$

This shows that a two-dimensional inverse Fourier transform of the k-space data $S(k_x, k_y)$ gives $\rho(x,y)$, in other words the MR image, as shown in Figure 5.22. In fact, the inverse Fourier transform gives a complex image, with real and imaginary components, but MR images are nearly always represented in magnitude mode, i.e. the magnitude of the real and imaginary components. Also in Figure 5.22 it is clear that the maximum acquired signal occurs at the centre of k-space, $k_x = 0$, $k_y = 0$. This can be seen from Equation (5.31), in which both exponential terms become unity. The low values of k-space correspond to low spatial frequencies, with the value of k_{max} representing the highest spatial frequency, as discussed in Chapter 1. The higher is the value of k_{max}, i.e. the higher the number of phase encoding steps acquired, the higher the spatial resolution.

5.11 Multiple-slice imaging

The imaging sequence shown in Figure 5.15 acquires an image from one slice through the body. Clearly, one would like to acquire images from multiple slices through the patient. If it were necessary to repeat this process serially for every single slice, then MR scanning would take an extremely long time. As noted earlier, the typical T_2^* values for tissue are much shorter than the T_1 relaxation times, and so the TR time required between successive RF excitations for each phase encoding step is much longer than the TE. Therefore, the 'waiting time', TR-TE, can be used to acquire data from other slices. To excite a slice exactly adjacent to the previous one, the only parameter that needs to be changed is the centre frequency of the RF pulse: the slice select, phase and frequency encoding gradients are repeated exactly as before, and the data from this second slice are stored separately from the first. This process is shown in Figure 5.23. The maximum number of slices is given by the value of TR/TE. In practice, a small gap is left between the slices (typically one-tenth of the slice thickness) and the slices are acquired in an interlaced fashion, i.e. all the odd-numbered slices followed by all the even-numbered. The reason is that the non-ideal frequency profile of the RF

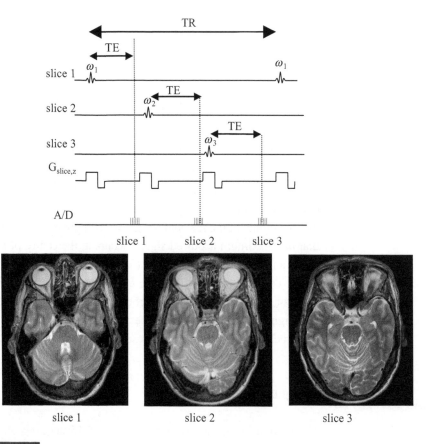

Figure 5.23

(top) Multiple-slice gradient echo sequence, which can be used to acquire many adjacent slices during one TR interval. For clarity, only the slice select gradient is shown: in practice the phase encoding and frequency encoding gradients are applied according to Figure 5.15(b) for each slice in turn. (bottom) Three adjacent axial slices through the brain acquired with the slice select direction being in z.

pulses results in a small angle tip of the protons either side of the selected slice. By waiting a time TR/2 to acquire these adjacent slices, the magnetization outside each slice has time to return to its full equilibrium value.

5.12 Basic imaging sequences

A typical clinical MRI protocol takes between half-an-hour and an hour, and may consist of between three and six different types of scan. The following sections cover the basic sequences used in most clinical scans: more advanced concepts are expanded upon in Section 5.16.

5.12.1 Multi-slice gradient echo sequences

The basic gradient echo sequence has already been analyzed in Section 5.8, with the imaging sequence shown in Figure 5.15. For an axial image acquired using slice-selection in the z-direction, the image intensity of each (x,y) voxel, I(x,y), is given by:

$$I(x, y) \propto \rho(x, y) \frac{\left(1 - e^{-\frac{TR}{T_1}}\right) \sin \alpha}{1 - e^{-\frac{TR}{T_1}} \cos \alpha} e^{-\frac{TE}{T_2^*}}. \tag{5.34}$$

Although the SNR is maximized using $\alpha = 90°$, this requires a long TR to allow full T_1 relaxation to occur, and in turn gives rise to a long image acquisition time. For example, if the tissue T_1 is 1 s, and TR is set to $3*T_1$ to allow almost complete (>95%) T_1 relaxation, then a 256×256 multi-slice image data set will take 8 minutes to acquire, and a high resolution 512×512 over 16 minutes, which is extremely long by clinical standards.

To image more rapidly, α is reduced to a value considerably smaller than 90°. It is relatively easy to show (Exercise 5.11) that for a given value of TR the value of α which maximizes the signal intensity is given by

$$\alpha_{Ernst} = \cos^{-1} e^{-\frac{TR}{T_1}}. \tag{5.35}$$

where the optimal angle, α_{Ernst} is named after the Swiss scientist Richard Ernst who won the Nobel Prize for Chemistry in 1989 for his contributions to magnetic resonance. For example, if TR is reduced to $0.05\ T_1$ then the optimum value of α is only 8°. Using these parameters, images can be acquired in a few tens of seconds.

Example 5.6 For a TR time equal to the T_1 value of the tissue, what angle should used for the RF pulse to maximize the SNR? How much greater is the SNR than would have been achieved had the RF pulse mistakenly been set to 90°?

Solution The optimal angle is given by:

$$\alpha_{Ernst} = \cos^{-1} e^{-1} = \cos^{-1}(0.3679) = 68°.$$

Plugging this value into Equation (5.34) gives an I(x,y) value of $0.68\rho(x,y)e^{-TE/T2}$. If an angle of 90° had been used, then this value would have been $0.63\,\rho(x,y)e^{-TE/T2}$.

From Equation (5.34) one can see that there are three separate components that affect the signal intensity: the proton density, a combination of the TR, T_1 and α values, and the TE and T_2* values. The data acquisition parameters in a gradient-echo sequence can be set to emphasize, or 'weight', the image intensity by one or all of the tissue parameters $\rho(x,y)$, T_1 or T_2*, depending upon the choice of data acquisition parameters. For example, suppose that we are trying to differentiate between two tissues A and B. The proton density for A is 1.0, and for B is 1.2. The T_1 value for A is 1 s and that of B is 1.3 s. Finally, the T_2* of A is 35 ms, and of B is 30 ms. If the value of TE is set to 1 ms, then the relative signals due to T_2* decay *alone* are 0.972 and 0.967 for A and B respectively, a very small difference. Therefore, the image intensity is not 'weighted' by the different values of T_2* for tissues A and B. In contrast, if TE is set to 30 ms, then the signals are 0.368 and 0.424 which is a much larger difference: the image can now be said to be T_2*-weighted. Similarly, for a given value of TR, the higher the value of α the higher the T_1-weighting of the image, i.e. the greater the extent to which the relative intensities of tissues A and B depend upon the respective T_1 values. Alternatively, for a fixed α the shorter the TR the higher is the T_1-weighting. Finally, the proton density of course cannot be changed, since it is a fixed physical value. If the sequence parameters are chosen so that there is no T_1-weighting and no T_2*-weighting, then the image is said to be proton-density weighted. Table 5.2 shows the possible combinations of imaging parameters and the corresponding weighting.

5.12.2 Spin echo sequences

Gradient-echo sequences allow very rapid image acquisition. The major disadvantage is that they do not allow images to be weighted by the different T_2 values, but rather only by the T_2* value. Since, as discussed previously, T_2* values are typically much shorter than T_2 this leads not only to lower signal intensities than if one

Table 5.2: Relationship between imaging parameters and image weighting for a gradient-echo imaging sequence

Imaging parameters	Image weighting
TE $\ll T_2^*$, and either $\alpha \ll \alpha_{Ernst}$ or TR $\gg T_1$ or both	proton density
TE $\ll T_2^*$, and either $\alpha \sim \alpha_{Ernst}$ or TR $\sim T_1$ or both	T_1-weighted
TE $> T_2^*$, and either $\alpha \ll \alpha_{Ernst}$ or TR $\gg T_1$ or both	T_2^*-weighted
TE $> T_2^*$, and either $\alpha \sim \alpha_{Ernst}$ or TR $\sim T_1$ or both	mixed T_1- and T_2^*-weighted

could weight by T_2, but also the differences in the tissue T_2 values can be 'masked' by the much larger effects that lead to T_2^* decay. So tissues with quite different T_2 values may have much more similar T_2^* values since these are affected by magnet and tissue inhomogeneities. To introduce pure T_2-contrast into the image, a second class of sequences is used, termed spin-echo sequences [6].

In a spin-echo sequence two RF pulses are used, the first 90° pulse creates M_y magnetization, and the second 180° pulse refocuses the effects of T_2^+ relaxation. In order to see how the sequence works, first consider the effects of the RF pulses only as shown in Figure 5.24. Immediately succeeding the 90° pulse the M_y component is equal to M_0. The effect of T_2^+, as shown in Section 5.5, is to cause protons to have slightly different frequencies, denoted here as $\Delta\omega$, and the net magnetization vector decreases. At a time τ after the 90° pulse, each proton has precessed through an angle φ, given by $\varphi = (\Delta\omega)\tau$, and has components of both M_x and M_y magnetization related by:

$$\varphi = \arctan\left(\frac{M_x}{M_y}\right). \tag{5.36}$$

The 180° pulse applied about the x-axis does not affect the M_x component of magnetization, but converts the M_y component into $- M_y$. The effect, from Equation (5.34), is to convert the phase of the magnetization from $+ \varphi°$ to $(180 - \varphi)°$, as shown in Figure 5.24. During the second τ interval, the precessing magnetization accumulates an additional phase $+ \varphi$, and so the total phase is 180°, meaning that all vectors lie along the $- y$ axis, and the signal loss during the time 2τ is due to T_2 relaxation alone. Since the rephasing of the vectors does not depend upon the value of $\Delta\omega$, the effects of T_2^+ are cancelled for all protons:

$$S(2\tau) \propto M_0 e^{-\frac{2\tau}{T_2}}. \tag{5.37}$$

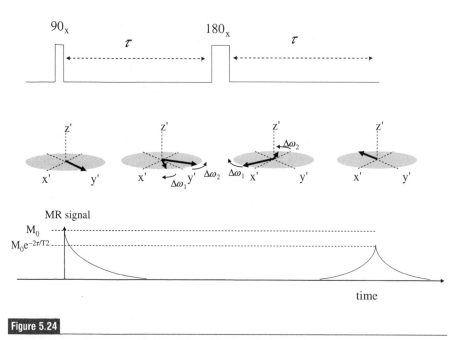

Spin echo sequence consisting of two RF pulses separated by a time τ. During this τ interval, protons precess at slightly different frequencies (two protons are shown with frequencies $\Delta\omega_1$ and $\Delta\omega_2$ with respect to the Larmor frequency) due to inhomogeneities in the main magnetic field (T_2^+) and intrinsic T_2 mechanisms. The effect of the 180° pulse is to refocus the T_2^+ decay, so that the intensity of the echo signal acquired at a time τ after the 180° pulse is affected only by T_2 processes.

In the imaging version of the spin-echo sequence, shown in Figure 5.25, the 90° and 180° pulses are applied together with G_{slice} to select and refocus protons in the desired slice. Phase-encoding is carried out exactly as described previously for the gradient-echo sequence. In the frequency encoding dimension, the dephasing gradient in a spin-echo sequence is applied between the 90° and 180° pulses with the same polarity as is used during data acquisition.

The intensity of an axial image acquired using a spin-echo sequence is given by:

$$I(x, y) \propto \rho(x, y)\left(1 - e^{-\frac{TR}{T_1}}\right)e^{-\frac{TE}{T_2}}. \tag{5.38}$$

Following the same type of analysis as in Section 5.11 for the gradient-echo sequence, a spin-echo image can be T_1-, T_2- or proton density-weighted. If the value of TR is set to a value much greater than or much less than the T_1 of any of the tissues, then the image has no T_1-weighting, since the term 1-exp(-TR/T_1) is very close to either unity or zero for all tissues. The general concept is shown in Figure 5.26, using T_1 values of 900 ms for grey and 780 ms for white matter. There is an optimal value of TR which maximizes the contrast between white and grey

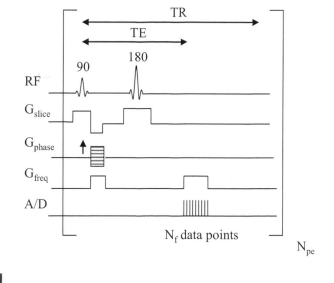

Figure 5.25

Basic spin echo imaging sequence.

matter. The same type of consideration applies to the term $\exp(-TE/T_2)$ in Equation (5.38) which determines the degree of 'T$_2$-weighting' in the sequence. If the value of TE is set to be much shorter than the tissue T_2 values, then no T_2 contrast is present, and if the value of TE is too long, then the SNR of the image is very low: the optimum value of TE results in the highest image CNR, as shown in Figure 5.26.

Images can also be acquired with 'proton-density-weighting' by setting a TR value much longer than T_1, and a TE value much shorter than T_2. Multi-slice imaging is performed in exactly the same way as for gradient-echo imaging. Figure 5.27 shows spin-echo images of the brain with different contrast weightings.

5.12.3 Three-dimensional imaging sequences

In multiple-slice gradient-echo or spin-echo imaging sequences, the in-plane image resolution is typically much higher than the slice thickness. For example, the slice thickness for a typical brain scan might be 3 mm, but the in-plane resolution is given by the image field-of-view (~25 cm) divided by the number of data points acquired (256 or 512) i.e. 1 or 0.5 mm. In situations where an isotropic high spatial resolution is needed, a three-dimensional sequence can be run: a 3D gradient-echo sequence is shown in Figure 5.28. There are now two phase encoding gradients, each of which must be incremented independently of the

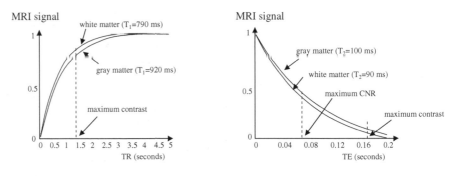

Figure 5.26

(left) Plot of MRI signal as a function of TR for white and grey matter in the brain at 1.5 Tesla. The maximum contrast occurs at a TR value of ~1.4 s, with the contrast-to-noise also maximized very close to this value. (right) Plot of MRI signal vs. TE for white and grey matter. In this case the maximum contrast occurs at a long value of TE, but because the signal intensity has decayed to a very low value by this point, the maximum CNR actually occurs at a somewhat shorter TE value.

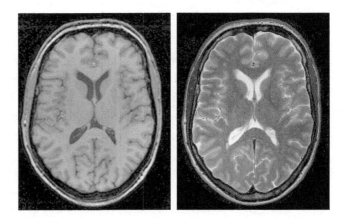

Figure 5.27

(left) T_1-weighted and (right) T_2-weighted axial slice through the brain acquired with a spin-echo sequence. In the T_1-weighted image the CSF filling the ventricles is much darker than the brain white/grey matter, whereas in the T_2-weighted image it is much brighter.

other. This means that the total imaging time is $TR \times N_{pe1} \times N_{pe2}$. For the total acquisition time to be practical within a clinical setting, the TR must be very short, meaning that most 3D sequences are gradient-echo based. Mathematically, the 3D acquired signal can be represented as:

$$S(k_x, k_y, k_z) = \int_{-\infty}^{\infty} \int_{-\infty}^{\infty} \int_{-\infty}^{\infty} \rho(x, y, z) e^{-j2\pi(k_x x + k_y y + k_z z)} dk_x dk_y dk_z. \quad (5.39)$$

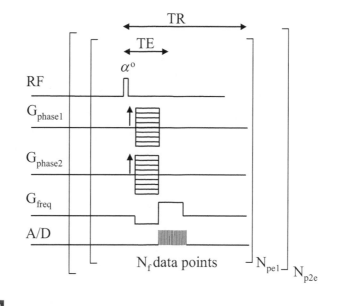

Figure 5.28

Three-dimensional gradient echo sequence. There are two incremental phase encoding gradients and one frequency encoding gradient.

Image reconstruction, therefore, uses a three-dimensional inverse Fourier transform. In addition to enabling high spatial resolution in all three dimensions, the 3D sequence is very efficient since signal is acquired from the entire imaging volume for every step in the acquisition, as opposed to just a single slice each time for a 2D multi-slice sequence.

5.13 Tissue relaxation times

As seen in Table 5.1, the T_1 and T_2 relaxation times can be quite different for tissues such as cerebral spinal fluid (CSF), kidney and liver, but are quite similar for grey and white brain matter. The relaxation times can be related to the general physical properties of the tissue, as well as to chemical properties such as iron and protein content. Intuitively, one can understand that just as application of a magnetic field oscillating at the Larmor frequency (the RF pulse) was required to establish a nonequilibrium M_z value, re-establishment of the equilibrium value of M_z must occur via a similar mechanism. The oscillating magnetic field which produces relaxation is not created by an RF pulse, but rather by the random Brownian motion of the magnetic moments in tissue. These randomly fluctuating magnetic fields contain components at many different frequencies: a fluid liquid such as CSF has a broad range of frequencies from very low to very high, whereas a tissue such as cartilage in which the protons are held in a very tight matrix can produce only low frequencies. The 'frequency spread' of the oscillating magnetic fields is quantified by a parameter called the spectral density, $J(\omega)$ or $J(f)$. The higher the value of $J(f)$, the greater the oscillating magnetic field component at that frequency. The component of $J(f)$ at the Larmor frequency, $J(f_0)$, can stimulate transitions between the upper and lower energy states, and thereby cause the M_z component of magnetization to return to its equilibrium value of M_0. The larger the value of $J(f_0)$, therefore, the more effective is the T_1 relaxation process and the shorter the T_1 relaxation time.

Figure 5.29 shows typical plots of $J(f)$ vs. frequency, with three specific clinical B_0 fields highlighted. Three different tissue types are indicated: one very viscous such as cartilage, one of intermediate viscosity such as brain grey matter, and one highly fluid such as the CSF in the brain. The general shapes of the curves for the three tissues are quite similar. At low magnetic fields the plots are flat, with a significant decrease in $J(f)$ only occurring at ~1.5 Tesla for the cartilage and above 4 Tesla for the CSF. From Figure 5.29 one can deduce that the T_1 relaxation time for all tissues increases as a function of field strength, but that this increase is highly non-linear. At low magnetic fields, T_1 relaxation for

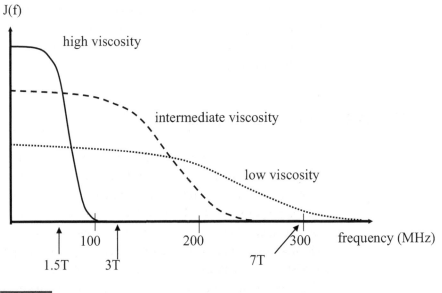

Figure 5.29

Plot of spectral density, J(f), vs. frequency for three tissue viscosities. Also marked are the resonant frequencies at three common magnetic field strengths, 1.5 Tesla (63.9 MHz), 3 Tesla (127.7 MHz) and 7 Tesla (298.1 MHz).

the cartilage is very efficient since the value of J(f) is high and therefore the T_1 value is short. At high field strengths, T_1 relaxation for cartilage is very inefficient and the T_1 value is long. Figure 5.29 also shows that the best contrast between the three tissues occurs at low magnetic field strengths, and that at very high magnetic fields all tissues have similar and high values of T_1. However, of course, the MR signal intensity is much lower at very low field strengths, representing a trade-off between image contrast and SNR in terms of the value of B_0.

The dependence of T_2 on field strength is more complicated. The value of $J(f_0)$ also contributes to T_2 relaxation, but there is an extra contribution to T_2 relaxation which is caused by local magnetic field fluctuations that occur at very low frequencies, i.e. the value of $J(f = 0)$. The result is that T_2 is always shorter than T_1. In cartilage, the high value of $J(f = 0)$ means that T_2 is very short. As noted earlier, there is no direct relationship between the T_1 and T_2 of a tissue at a given field strength.

5.14 MRI instrumentation

There are three major hardware components which constitute the MRI scanner: the magnet, an RF coil and three magnetic field gradient coils. As has been described previously, the magnet produces a net magnetization within the patient, the RF coil produces the pulse of magnetic energy required to create transverse magnetization and also receives the MRI signal via Faraday induction, and the magnetic field gradient coils impose a linear variation on the proton resonance frequency as a function of position in each of the three spatial dimensions.

In addition to these three components, there are electronic circuits used to turn the gradients on and off, to produce RF pulses of pre-determined length and amplitude, and to amplify and digitize the signal. A block diagram of a simplified MRI system is shown in Figure 5.30.

5.14.1 Superconducting magnet design

The vast majority of MRI magnets are superconducting. Since the early 2000s many 1.5 Tesla scanners have been replaced by 3 Tesla systems, with almost universally better image quality. As outlined in Section 5.4, the MRI signal increases as the square of the B_0 field. Commercial human-sized magnets have also been produced at 7 Tesla and 9.4 Tesla but are not yet in routine clinical use.

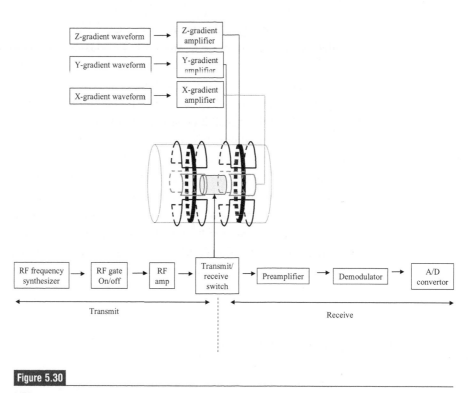

Figure 5.30

MRI system hardware components used to control the gradients and RF transmitter and receiver. Each gradient has a separate waveform and amplifier. The transmit and receive sides of the RF chain are separated by a transmit/receive switch.

The two major aims of magnet design are: (i) to produce the most homogeneous magnetic field over the sample to give the longest T_2^* relaxation time, and (ii) to produce a stable magnetic field in which the drift is of the order of 1 part per billion (1 ppb) over the course of an MRI scan.

The basis of creating a strong magnetic field is to pass high current through a series of coils of conducting wire. The most commonly used geometry is based on a solenoid, or helix. For a long solenoid, the magnetic field is very homogeneous over the central part of the solenoid. At the centre, the value of the magnetic field is given by:

$$B = \frac{\mu_0 nI}{\sqrt{L^2 + 4R^2}}, \tag{5.40}$$

where μ_0 is the permeability of free space (1.257×10^{-6} T mA^{-1}), n is the number of turns, I is the current passing through the wires, L is the length of the solenoid and R is the radius of the solenoid.

Example 5.7   Calculate the required current to produce a magnetic field of 3 Tesla using values of R = 50 cm, L = 1.5 m, and 100 turns of wire per cm.

Solution   The total number of turns of wire is 15 000, using very thin wire! Substituting into Equation (5.40):

$$3(\text{T}) = \frac{1.257\text{x}10^{-6}(\text{TmA}^{-1})15000\text{I}(\text{A})}{\sqrt{1.5 + 1}(\text{m})}$$

gives a current of 250 A.

As suggested by the numerical example above, the problem in using simple copper wire is the immense amount of heat that is created by passing a very large current through such a solenoid. The power deposited is proportional to the square of the current multiplied by the resistance of the wire. To reduce the heat dissipation, the resistance of the wire needs to be made extremely low, and this leads to the use of superconducting wire. Certain materials exhibit zero resistance at very low temperatures, a phenomenon known as superconductivity. For MRI magnets, these wires must be capable of carrying several hundreds of amps, and of remaining superconducting within the strong magnetic field that the wires themselves create.

The most commonly used material for superconducting wires is an alloy of niobium-titanium. The alloy is very flexible and is formed into multi-stranded filaments which are distributed within a copper matrix to form a flexible wire. Although a simple solenoid produces a reasonably homogeneous magnetic field, it can be improved by increasing the number of solenoids, and varying their positions and diameters, as shown in Figure 5.31. The standard number of solenoids is six, although some magnet designs have up to ten. The wires are wound in recessed slots in aluminium formers and are fixed in place using epoxy adhesive. The entire windings are housed in a stainless steel can, called the cryostat, which contains liquid helium at a temperature of 4.2 K, as shown in Figure 5.31. This can is surrounded by a series of radiation shields and vacuum vessels to minimize the boil-off of the liquid helium. The radiation shields are themselves cooled by cryogenic refrigerators based on the Gifford-McMahon cycle. In older magnets, an outer container of liquid nitrogen is used to cool the outside of the vacuum chamber and the radiation shields: in more modern systems compressed helium gas is circulated by a cold head and cools the outer radiation shield. Since gas losses cannot be completely eliminated, liquid helium must be replenished, typically on an annual basis.

The magnet is energized by passing current (typically 100–300 A) into the major filament windings. Since the wire is superconducting, after 'energizing' the

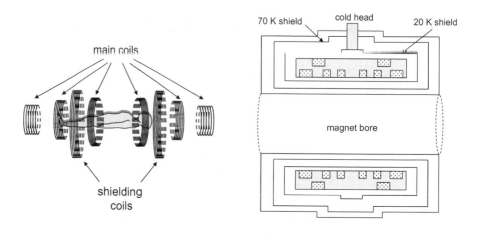

main coils

shielding
coils

70 K shield   cold head   20 K shield

magnet bore

Figure 5.31

(left) The solenoidal coils used to produce a homogeneous static magnetic field. Six solenoids (main coils) are positioned along the z-axis. Two shielding coils are used to reduce the effect of the 'stray field' outside the magnet. (right) Cutaway of a superconducting magnet. The grey tinted areas represent those filled with liquid helium to make the wires superconducting. Two aluminium radiation shields are kept at 20 K and 70 K.

magnet, the power source is removed and the current circulates through the magnet essentially indefinitely. Fine tuning of the magnet homogeneity is performed by using a series of independent superconducting coils, termed shim coils, to reach the manufacturer's specifications. There is also a set of room temperature shim coils that are used to optimize the homogeneity for each clinical scan, depending upon the particular organ being imaged and the individual patient. This is normally performed automatically during scan preparation.

The final issue with the superconducting magnet is siting. There is typically a very large 'fringe field' which extends well outside the magnet itself. Since most electronic equipment cannot operate in strong magnetic fields, and these fields also pose hazards for people with pacemakers, there is effectively a large wasted space around the magnet. One solution is to actively shield the magnet, in other words to add secondary shielding coils as shown in Figure 5.31, which are specifically designed to minimize the stray field outside the magnet via field cancellation. Alternatively, passive shielding in the form of annealed low-carbon steel can be added to the room in which the magnet is situated in order to confine the stray magnetic field.

5.14.2 Magnetic field gradient coils

As shown in Figure 5.30, three separate gradient coils are each fed by a separate gradient amplifier. The current (up to several hundred amps) from each amplifier can be switched on and off in less than 1 ms. The maximum gradient strength depends upon the maximum current that can be passed through the gradient coils without causing excessive heating. The gradient coils are constructed of copper and are usually water-cooled. They are wound on cylindrical formers, which are bolted to the inner bore of the magnet. Currents passing through the coils cause alternating Lorenz forces within the magnetic field, and these forces must be balanced to avoid putting a large strain on the gradients. In fact, the loud sound of an MRI scan results from the whole cylinder vibrating, and these vibrations being translated to very complicated motions of the other components within the MRI system through mechanical contact [7]. Acoustic damping is used, but the sound levels are still well above 100 dB and so the use of earplugs and headphones is mandatory.

The aims in gradient coil design are: (i) to produce the maximum gradient per unit current, (ii) to minimize the 'rise' time of the gradient, i.e. how fast it can reach its prescribed value, and (iii) to achieve the maximum volume of gradient linearity, usually defined as being 95% of the value in the exact centre of the gradient coil. Very simple designs, such as are shown in Figure 5.32, can be derived from analytical expressions for the magnetic fields created by loops of wire. The simplest configuration for the coil producing a gradient in the z-direction is a 'Maxwell pair', shown on the left of Figure 5.32, which consists of two loops each consisting of multiple turns of wire. The two loops are wound in opposite directions around a cylindrical former, and the loops are spaced by a separation of $\sqrt{3}$ times the radius

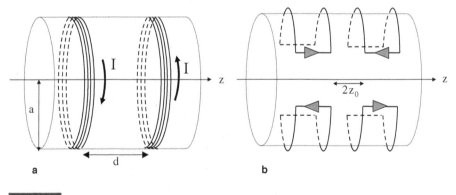

Figure 5.32

(a) Basic geometry of a Maxwell-pair gradient coil which produces a magnetic field gradient in the z-direction. The two halves consist of equal numbers of turns of wire, with equal currents in each half but flowing in opposite directions. The magnetic fields from the two halves cancel in the centre of the gradient set. In the configuration shown, the left-hand half produces a magnetic field opposite to B_0 (using Fleming's left-hand rule) and therefore the resonant frequency increases in the positive z-direction. (b) Basic saddle-geometry for producing a transverse gradient, in this case in the y-direction. The direction of current in the four identical components of the gradient coil is indicated by the arrows. The design for producing an x-gradient is the same, but rotated by 90°.

of each loop. The magnetic field produced by this gradient coil is zero at the centre of the coil, and is linearly dependent upon position in the z-direction over about one-third of the separation of the two loops. For loops of radius a, the gradient efficiency, η, is given by:

$$\eta = \frac{8.058 \times 10^{-7} nI}{a^2} \, Tm^{-1}, \tag{5.41}$$

where n is the number of turns, and I is the current through the wires.

The x- and y-gradient coils are completely independent of the z-gradient coils, and are connected to two separate gradient amplifiers. From symmetry considerations the same basic design can be used for coils producing gradients in the x- and y-directions with the geometries simply rotated by 90°. The simplest configuration is the 'saddle coil' arrangement, with four arcs, as shown on the right of Figure 5.32. Each arc subtends an angle of 120°, the separation between the arcs along the z-axis is 0.8 times the radius of the gradient coil, and the length of each arc is 2.57 times the radius. The efficiency of this design is given by:

$$\eta = \frac{9.18 \times 10^{-7} nI}{a^2} \, Tm^{-1}. \tag{5.42}$$

The three criteria (homogeneity, switching speed and efficiency) for judging gradient performance can be combined into a so-called figure-of-merit, β, defined as [8]:

$$\beta = \frac{\eta^2}{L\sqrt{\frac{1}{V} \int \left(\frac{B(r)}{B_0(r)} - 1\right)^2 d^3r}}, \tag{5.43}$$

where L is the inductance of the coil, $B_0(r)$ is the 'desired' magnetic field and B(r) is the actual magnetic field, and V is the volume of interest over which the integral is evaluated. More sophisticated geometries than the simple saddle-shaped coils have been designed, based upon numerical optimization schemes, to increase the figure-of-merit. An example is shown in Figure 5.33: because of their design these are termed 'fingerprint coils' [9].

When current in the gradient coils is switched rapidly, eddy currents can be induced in nearby conducting surfaces such as the radiation shield in the magnet. These eddy currents, in turn, produce additional unwanted gradients which may decay only very slowly even after the original gradients have been switched off: these eddy currents can result in significant image artifacts. All gradient coils in commercial MRI systems are now 'actively shielded' [10] to reduce the effects of eddy currents. Active shielding uses a second set of coils placed outside the main gradient coils, the effect of which is to minimize the stray gradient fields.

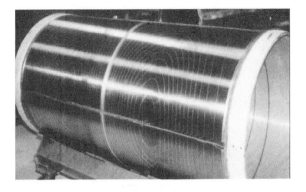

A fingerprint gradient set, used to produce a y-gradient. The design is usually milled from a solid piece of copper and mounted on to a fibre-glass cylindrical former, which is then securely bolted on to the inside of the magnet bore.

5.14.3 Radiofrequency coils

The dual role of the RF coil is to transmit pulses of RF energy into the body, and also to detect the precessing magnetization via Faraday induction. Since the frequencies of transmission and reception are the same, a single RF coil can be used to perform both tasks. However, more commonly, separate coils are used for transmission and reception, with an array of small coils usually being employed to receive the signal.

The basic coil is a 'tuned' RF circuit, designed to operate most efficiently at the Larmor frequency. The 'LC' circuit is one in which conductive elements form the inductor (L), and capacitance (C) is added in order to tune the coil to the appropriate frequency. The conductor is either copper or silver wire or tape, since these metals have the highest conductivity. The resonant frequency of the LC circuit is given by:

$$\omega_{\text{res}} \approx \frac{1}{\sqrt{\text{LC}}} \text{ or } f_{\text{res}} \approx \frac{1}{2\pi\sqrt{\text{LC}}}. \tag{5.44}$$

The coil is attached to the transmitter and receiver chain, shown in Figure 5.34, through coaxial cables which have a characteristic impedance of 50 Ω, and so for maximum power transfer the RF coil should also be impedance matched to this value. The most common circuit for 'tuning and matching' an RF coil to 50 Ω at the Larmor frequency is shown in Figure 5.34. The resistance shown in the circuit is that of the conductor used to make the coil.

The highest efficiency is achieved by matching the size of the RF coil as closely as possible to the size of the body part being imaged. In most systems (except for

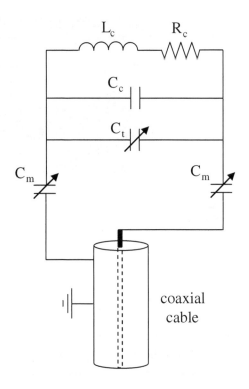

Figure 5.34

Basic electrical circuit used to impedance match the RF coil to 50 Ω at the Larmor frequency. The intrinsic inductance, capacitance and resistance of the RF coil are denoted by L_c, C_c and R_c, respectively. Three external capacitors (C_t and two equal value capacitors C_m) are connected to the RF coil to form the impedance matching network. The arrows denote that these can be variable capacitors whose value can be changed for each patient if required. The coil and impedance matching network are connected to the rest of the MRI system via a coaxial cable with 50 Ω impedance.

very high magnetic field strengths >7 Tesla) a large cylindrical body coil is integrated into the MRI system by being bolted on to the inside of the gradient set. This type of coil is used for abdominal imaging, for example. The larger the RF coil, the higher the power necessary, and for a body-coil at 3 Tesla the RF amplifier must be able to supply 30 kW of power at ~128 MHz. For smaller body parts such as the head and the knee, in which the whole 'organ' is to be imaged, a smaller cylindrical RF coil, as shown in Figure 5.35, is placed around the head or knee. Both the body coil and smaller volume coils in Figure 5.35 are designed to produce a spatially uniform B_1 field across the entire imaging volume. From electromagnetic theory, in order to achieve a very uniform field the required current density is proportional to the sine of the azimuthal angle of the cylindrical coil. A practical realization of this theoretical result is the 'birdcage coil' [11], which uses a large

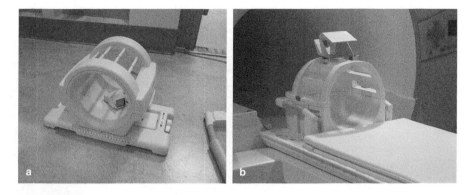

(a) A commercial knee coil for a 3 Tesla magnet, formed from twelve rungs in a birdcage geometry. The structure has an upper and lower half to facilitate patient positioning. (b) Similar structure for a head coil, with a mirror attached so that the patient can see out of the end of the magnet, which is useful if visual stimuli are needed for functional MRI experiments.

number of parallel conductors, typically between 16 and 32, as can be seen in the coils in Figure 5.35.

On the receive side, the MRI signal induced in the RF coil is of the order of tens of millivolts. Noise in the measurement comes predominantly from the resistance of the body which, being conducting and having current flowing through it, produces random voltages which are picked up by the coil. It is advantageous to cover the region of interest with a large number of smaller more sensitive coils, called a coil array. Each coil couples very closely to the body, but picks up noise only from a small part of the body. Overall, the signal-to-noise is improved significantly using this approach compared to having a single larger receive coil. Each of the small coils must be electrically isolated from the others, and the RF coils are usually geometrically overlapped to maximize this isolation, and in addition preamplifier decoupling also reduces the interaction between coils [12]. Figure 5.36 shows a large commercial perivascular array containing 24 separate receive coils. The signal from each coil is fed into a separate receive channel, before the signals are combined into a composite image.

It is also necessary, when having separate transmit and receive RF coils, that these are electrically decoupled from one another. Since they are tuned to the same frequency, if both are active at one time there will be interference between the RF coils and the efficiency will be much lower. Typically, actively-switched non-magnetic PIN diodes are used to decouple the coils [13]. For example, in Figure 5.37, the array of surface coils is detuned during transmission and tuned during signal reception. Using similar circuitry, the transmit coil is tuned during transmission and detuned during signal reception.

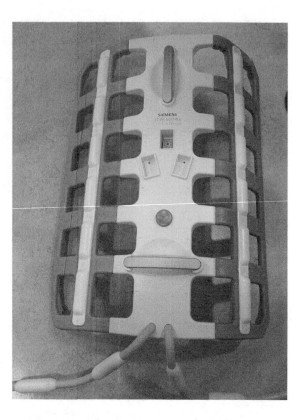

Figure 5.36

Multi-element body array for 3 Tesla consisting of 24 separate elements. Each element is electrically decoupled from the other individual elements. The array is used to receive the MR signal, with a large body coil which is fixed inside the bore of the magnet used to transmit the RF pulses.

As shown in Figure 5.30, the transmit and receive sections are separated by a transmit/receive switch. This is required to protect the receive side from the very high power pulses during RF transmission (which would otherwise literally destroy the receiver) and also to route all of the MR signal to the receiver rather than back to the transmitter. The transmit/receive switch must be capable of handling very high power, be able to switch in microseconds, and have excellent isolation between the two channels.

5.14.4 Receiver design

The small voltages induced in the receive coils are amplified by a high-gain low-noise preamplifier. These signals are then demodulated to a lower frequency (using circuitry very similar to a conventional FM radio) and

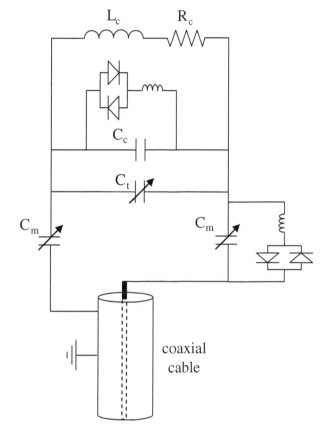

Figure 5.37

A circuit that can be used to decouple a receive coil (shown) from a transmit coil. When the transmit coil produces an RF pulse, a DC signal is sent to the diodes to make them conduct. This introduces two extra inductances into the circuit, each one producing a parallel circuit with the matching capacitors, C_m. If the value of the inductance is chosen correctly, then this forms two circuits with infinite impedance, and therefore the coil is no longer resonant. When the receiver coils are required to be active to acquire the signal, the DC signal is turned off, the diodes become non-conducting and the receiver resonant circuit is re-established.

digitized, typically at a sampling rate of 80 MHz with a resolution of 14-bits. Since this bandwidth is much higher than actually required for the imaging experiment (see Example 5.8), after various corrections for gradient non-linearities, the raw digitized signal is decimated and filtered using a digital filter to the correct bandwidth as covered in Section 1.7, which describes the advantages of oversampling. These signals are then stored in memory and inverse Fourier transformed to give the MR image, displayed in magnitude mode. If a coil array is used, then the signals from each coil are stored separately and either combined to form the image, or undergo further processing if parallel imaging techniques are being used to speed up data acquisition, as described in the next section.

Example 5.8   A 3 Tesla image is being taken of the head, which has a dimension in the frequency-encoding direction of 25 cm. If the maximum gradient strength of 40 mT/m is used while the signal is being detected, what bandwidth must be used?

Solution   The bandwidth is given by 40 mT/m $\times$ 0.25 = 0.01 T. Since 1T = 42.58 MHz the bandwidth in Hz is given by ~425 kHz.

5.15 Parallel imaging using coil arrays

Perhaps the greatest technological breakthrough in the past ten years in MRI has been the development of parallel imaging techniques, which allow images to be acquired much more quickly by only acquiring a certain fraction (typically between one-quarter and one-half) of the k-space data. The ultimate limit to the speed of image acquisition is the rate at which the gradients can be switched on-and-off: this imposes a physical limit on the value of TR, and therefore on the total imaging time for a given spatial resolution in the phase encoding direction. For a given hardware set-up, the only way to increase imaging speed, while maintaining spatial resolution, is to reduce the extent of k-space coverage. For example, one might decide to acquire only every other phase encoding step: however, as shown in Figure 5.38 this causes unacceptable aliasing of the image (see Exercise 5.15).

The key concept in parallel imaging was to realize that, when an array of receive coils is used to acquire the image, there is already some spatial information available related to the signals acquired by each coil, i.e. coils close to a particular part of the body will receive signal from that part only, and not from an area on the opposite side of the body. Algorithms used for parallel imaging are mathematically complicated, and so only an intuitive explanation is given here: details can be found in the original references [14–17]. The simplest case is shown in Figure 5.39: in this case the head is being imaged with the signal acquired by two receiver coils, each one of which 'sees' only one-half of the brain, either the top- or bottom-half. In this case, the effect of only acquiring alternate lines in k_y is to stretch out the image in y for each coil, but since each coil only sees one half of the full field of view in the y-dimension, there is no aliasing of the image. From the two,

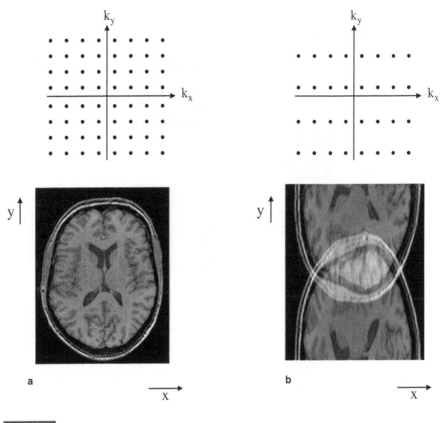

(a) A full k-space matrix (top) gives an unaliased image (bottom) provided that the Δk_x and Δk_y increments are correctly set. (b) If data acquisition speed is increased by a factor of 2 by acquiring only alternate k_y lines, then the Δk_y is doubled, the image field-of-view in the y-dimension is halved, and the image is aliased along the y-dimension.

non-overlapping stretched versions of the brain, it is very simple to add the images together and rescale to produce a full image, acquired in half the time of a fully encoded image.

The trade-off in parallel imaging is between the reduced data acquisition time and a reduced SNR. However, in many clinical situations the limiting factor is not the SNR but the time required to acquire an image. One example is abdominal imaging of the liver, in which it is important to be able to acquire the entire image within a single breath-hold to avoid image artifacts from motion. Clinical patients may only be able to hold their breath for less than ten seconds, and so rapid data acquisition is needed. An example is shown in Figure 5.40, in which dynamic swallowing of a water bolus is acquired in real-time using parallel imaging, which allowed a four-fold decrease in imaging time.

Full-encoded
images from
each coil

Half-encoded
images from
each coil

Combine

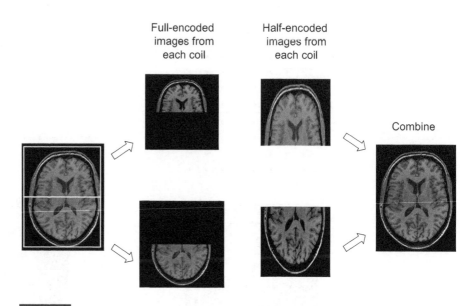

Figure 5.39

General principle of parallel imaging. Two RF coils, shown as white rectangles on the left, are used to acquire the MRI signal. If a full field-of-view image is acquired using full k-space encoding, then the two images from the two coils contain signal from either the top or bottom of the brain only. If only every other line of k-space is acquired, then the field of view in the y-dimension is halved, and so the images from each coil appear stretched, but are not aliased (unlike in Figure 5.38). Stitching together of the two images, and dimensional rescaling by a factor of two produces an unaliased image acquired in half the time of the fully encoded image.

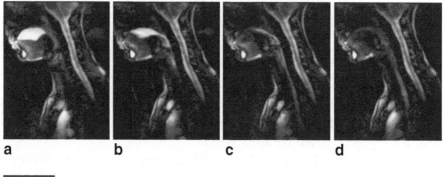

a   b   c   d

Figure 5.40

(a-d) Successive images from a subject who is swallowing water (bright signal). Data acquisition speed was increased four times over normal using parallel imaging.

5.16   Fast imaging sequences

In addition to the basic gradient-echo and spin-echo sequences covered previously, there are a large number of variations upon these basic ideas. In this section, two very rapid imaging sequences are covered, along with situations in which they are used.

5.16.1 Echo planar imaging

Multi-slice gradient-echo sequences can acquire image data sets from the entire brain, for example, in the order of tens of seconds when required. However, there are a small number of applications in which even faster imaging is called for. Such cases occur when a very large number of images must be acquired within a clinically-relevant timescale. One example is diffusion tensor imaging, in which case many tens of image datasets must be acquired using slightly different parameters for each dataset, with each dataset ideally covering the entire brain. A second example, covered in Section 5.18, is functional imaging in which many hundreds of different datasets must be acquired in a single session, again covering as much of the brain as possible.

As can be appreciated from the sequences covered so far, the major limitation in reducing the time for image acquisition is that the sequence must be repeated N_{pe} times, each time with a TR delay between successive RF excitations. In contrast, the fastest type of imaging sequence uses a single slice-selective RF pulse followed by sampling the whole of k-space before the signal has decayed due to T_2^* relaxation. These sequences are termed 'single-shot', since only a single excitation pulse is used to acquire the entire image. The most common sequence is echo-planar imaging (EPI), which can acquire a single slice 128×128 image in much less than 100 ms [18]. The simplest version of the EPI sequence is shown in Figure 5.41, together with the corresponding k-space sampling scheme.

Unlike conventional multi-slice imaging methodology, multi-slice EPI acquires the image from each slice sequentially, since there is no conventional TR delay. Since each slice can be acquired in ~50–100 ms depending upon the spatial resolution, whole-brain coverage can be achieved in ~1 s. The major disadvantage of the EPI sequence is that the signal decays between each successive phase encoding step, which introduces blurring in the phase encoding direction when the image is reconstructed. This is particularly true in areas with a very short T_2^*, such as at air/tissue interfaces. Here, a very short T_2^* can lead to signal voids, as well as significant image distortion artifacts. An example of this phenomenon is shown in Figure 5.42. To minimize this effect, while maintaining high imaging speed, the EPI sequence is often run in 'segmented-mode'. Segmented-EPI involves acquiring, for example, only every fourth line in k-space, and then repeating the sequence four times to acquire the full k-space matrix. In this way, the T_2^* relaxation during each of the four, interleaved acquisitions is much less

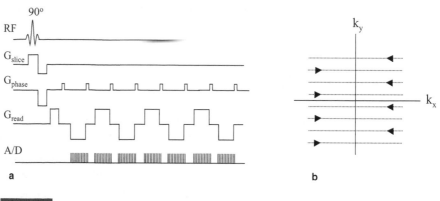

Figure 5.41

(a) Basic echo planar imaging sequence used for single-shot rapid MRI, and (b) Corresponding k-space coverage. The first data point acquired is at the maximum negative values of both k_x and k_y (bottom left) and proceeds according to the arrows, ending up at the maximum positive values of k_x and k_y (top right) via a zig-zag trajectory.

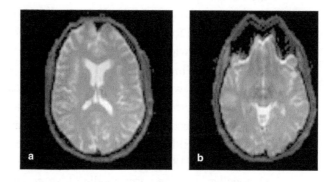

Figure 5.42

Two single-shot EPI images acquired in a patient's brain. Slice (a) was acquired in the middle of the brain, whereas slice (b) was acquired in an area close to the nasal cavities. The severe image distortions in (b) arise from the very short T_2^* values in brain tissue close to the tissue/air interface.

than in the single-shot implementation, and the image blurring effect is reduced significantly.

5.16.2 Turbo spin echo sequences

As outlined above, the major disadvantage of the EPI sequence is that the signal is weighted by T_2^* which can cause significant image distortions. These distortions can potentially be reduced by using a spin-echo rather than gradient-echo based sequence. To achieve a high imaging speed, multiple spin echoes rather than a

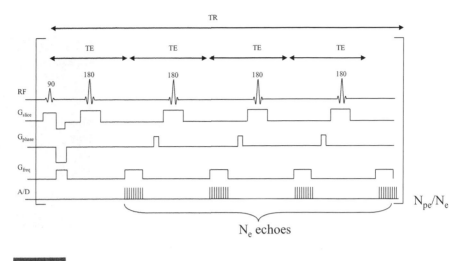

Turbo spin echo imaging sequence in which N_e echoes are acquired for each TR interval. This reduces the image acquisition time by a factor of N_e compared to a simple spin echo sequence.

single echo can be used: this type of sequence is called a turbo spin echo (TSE) sequence [19]. Figure 5.43 shows the basic imaging sequence, which can be considered as a hybrid of the EPI and spin-echo sequences.

Although it is technically possible to acquire 128 or 256 echoes and therefore the entire image in a single-shot, it is more common to acquire a smaller number of echoes, 16 or 32 is typical, and to acquire the image in a small number of shots, typically 8 or 16. A number of variations of this sequence exist, with slight differences in the way that the phase encoding gradient is applied, for example, but all are based on the basic principle shown in Figure 5.43. There is some image blurring in the phase encoding direction due to T_2 decay between successive phase encoding steps, but not as much as in a T_2^*-weighted sequence such as EPI. The major limitation of the TSE sequence, particularly at high magnetic fields, is the amount of energy deposited in the patient (see Section 5.21).

5.17 Magnetic resonance angiography

Unlike X-ray angiographic techniques covered in Chapter 2, magnetic resonance angiography (MRA) does not require the use of contrast agents, although they can be used to increase the signal difference between flowing blood and tissue. The most common technique is called time-of-flight (TOF) angiography [20], which is based on the much shorter effective T_1 ($T_{1,eff}$) of blood due to flow into and through the imaging slice if the slice (or volume) is oriented perpendicular to

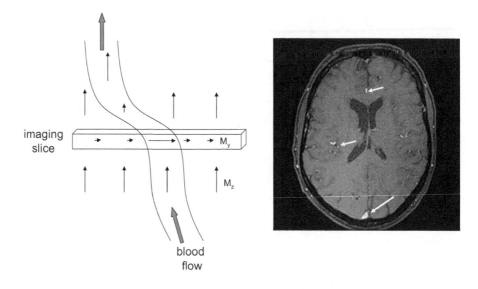

Figure 5.44

(left) The TOF MR angiographic technique. Blood flowing into the imaging slice has full M_z magnetization before the RF pulse, and so a 90° pulse creates maximum M_y magnetization. In contrast, stationary tissue within the slice experiences every RF pulse during the imaging sequence and since TR ≪ $3T_1$ is 'saturated', i.e. has an M_z magnetization which is much less than its thermal equilibrium value. Therefore, the 90° pulse creates a much lower M_y magnetization in the tissue than in the blood. (right) Image of a slice through the brain showing the vessels (arrows) with flow perpendicular to the image slice as bright spots.

the direction of flow, as shown in Figure 5.44. The actual T_1 value of the water in blood is similar to the value for many tissues. However, during the TR delay between successive RF pulses and phase encoding steps, a new pool of blood flows into the volume being imaged. These protons have not experienced any of the previous RF pulses and so if the slice is thin these protons have full magnetization ($M_z = M_0$). For a given slice thickness (S_{th}) and blood velocity (v), the value of $T_{1(eff)}$ of the blood is given by:

$$\frac{1}{T_{1(eff)}} = \frac{1}{T_1} + \frac{v}{S_{th}}. \tag{5.45}$$

For example, if the slice thickness is 5 mm, and a value of TR of 50 ms is used, blood flowing at speeds greater than 10 cm/s will flow completely out of the slice in the time between successive phase-encoding steps. The value of $T_{1(eff)}$ is therefore zero.

To differentiate between flowing blood and stationary tissue, a very heavily T_1-weighted sequence should be used with a high tip angle pulse (to get maximum signal from the blood) in combination with a short TR value (to minimize the

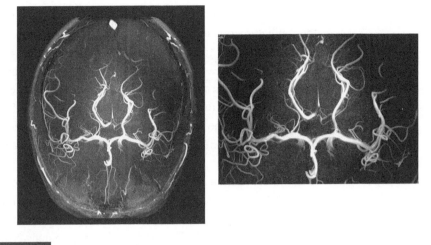

Figure 5.45

(left) Maximum intensity projection from a three-dimensional TOF sequence acquired in the brain. The circle-of-Willis is prominently shown close to the centre of the brain. (right) Expanded image shows the very fine and detailed vessel structure that can be obtained using MR angiography.

signal from the stationary tissue and acquire the data rapidly). The simplest implementation of the TOF principle uses a rapid gradient-echo sequence with a tip angle large compared to the Ernst angle for tissue.

Multi-slice or three-dimensional angiography is normally performed to obtain flow images throughout a given volume of the brain. A single image from a 3D data-set is shown on the right of Figure 5.44, with flowing blood showing up as the bright signal. The images are usually displayed using a maximum intensity projection (MIP) algorithm, as shown in Figure 5.45. For observation of very small vessels, contrast agents (see Section 5.19) can be used to reduce further the effective T_1 of blood, and increase the contrast between flowing spins and stationary tissue.

5.18 Functional MRI

Functional MRI (fMRI) is a technique to determine which areas of the brain are involved in specific cognitive tasks as well as general brain functions such as speech, language and sensory motion. The basis for the method is that the MRI signal intensity changes depending upon the level of oxygenation of the blood in the brain, a phenomenon termed the blood oxygen level dependent (BOLD) effect [21]. The level of oxygenation changes by small amounts in areas where neuronal activation occurs, as described below, and so these areas can be detected using MRI.

When neuronal activation occurs in the brain's grey matter the local blood flow in the capillary bed is increased and there is an increase in the blood oxygenation level, corresponding to a decrease in the concentration of deoxyhaemoglobin. Deoxyhaemoglobin has a magnetic susceptibility which is more paramagnetic than tissue and so the local magnetic field gradients between the blood in the capillary bed and tissue also decrease. As a result, the values of T_2 and T_2^* *increase* locally in areas of the brain which are associated with neuronal activation: the increase in MR signal on either T_2 or T_2^* weighted scans forms the basis of functional MRI .

The most common MR sequence used to collect the data is a multi-slice echo-planar imaging, since data acquisition is fast enough to obtain whole-brain coverage in a few seconds. Many different types of stimulus can be used: visual-, motor- or auditory-based. The changes in image intensity in activated areas are very small, typically only 0.2–2% using a 3 Tesla scanner, and so experiments are repeated a number of times with periods of rest (baseline) between each stimulation block. Data processing involves correlation of the MRI signal intensity for each pixel with the stimulation waveform, as shown in Figure 5.46, followed by statistical analysis to determine whether the correlation is significant. Typical scans may take 10–40 minutes, with several hundred repetitions of the stimulus/rest paradigm.

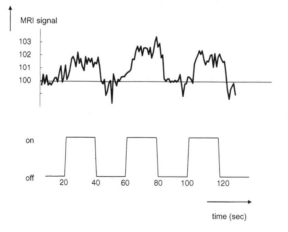
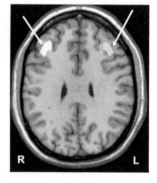

Figure 5.46

(left) Plot of the MR signal intensity within an activated voxel as a function of time, and below the time-course of the particular stimulus being presented. The MRI signal increase is delayed by approximately 6 s with respect to the stimulus due to the finite hemodynamic response time. Signal changes are of the order of a few percent. Correlation of the MRI signal intensity with the stimulus pattern on a pixel-by-pixel basis produces the voxels (right) which show a statistically significant correlation in two areas outlined by the arrows.

Although fMRI is currently used more for research than routine clinical use, it is increasingly being used in a number of presurgical planning studies. Here, the exact surgical 'route' for removing, for example, a tumour from the brain can be planned by avoiding areas which have been determined to be involved in critical cognitive tasks such as language recognition and motor processes.

5.19   MRI contrast agents

In many clinical scans, there is sufficient contrast-to-noise on the appropriate T_1-, T_2- or proton density-weighted image to distinguish diseased from healthy tissue. However, in certain cases such as the detection of very small lesions, where partial volume effects occur within the slice, the CNR may be too low for a definitive diagnosis. In this case, MRI contrast agents can be used to increase the CNR between healthy and diseased tissue. There are two basic classes of MRI contrast agent: paramagnetic and superparamagnetic, also called positive and negative agents, respectively. In addition to lesion detection, positive agents are also often used in combination with TOF angiography.

5.19.1   Positive contrast agents

Paramagnetic contrast agents shorten the T_1 of the tissue in which they accumulate, and are therefore referred to clinically as positive contrast agents since they increase the MRI signal on T_1-weighted scans. There are currently several different agents (which go by trade names such as Omniscan, Prohance and Magnevist) which are approved worldwide for clinical use. The differences between the various agents are in the ionicity and osmolarity, similar to X-ray contrast agents covered in Chapter 2. All the agents are based on a central gadolinium ion, which is surrounded by a particular chemical chelate, as shown in Figure 5.47. Neither the gadolinium nor the chelate produces an MR signal directly, but the chelated molecule is visualized via its effect on water molecules in the tissue in which the contrast agent accumulates. The Gd^{3+} ion has seven unpaired electrons, and the interaction between water protons and these electrons produces a very efficient T_1 relaxation and so reduces the T_1 time of the tissue. The agents are designed so that there is one empty binding site to the Gd ion which is not occupied by the chelate structure. This means that a water molecule can temporarily bind to this site, undergo very rapid T_1 relaxation and then be released to be succeeded by a second water molecule, and so on. This mechanism is referred to as 'inner sphere relaxation'. A second way in which water molecules can have their T_1 relaxation time reduced is simply by interacting with the unpaired Gd electrons at a distance,

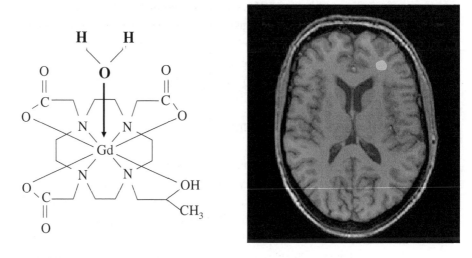

Figure 5.47

(left) The chemical structure of a positive MRI contrast agent (Prohance). One co-ordination position is free, which allows water to bind strongly but reversibly to the Gd-ion and undergo extremely fast T_1 relaxation. (right) One slice through the brain showing accumulation of the agent in a small lesion, which appears bright on a T_1-weighted sequence.

i.e. by diffusing close to the molecule: this latter mechanism is called 'outer sphere' relaxation and is not as efficient as inner sphere relaxation but many more water molecules are affected.

Gd-based paramagnetic contrast agents are most often used in the diagnosis of central nervous system (CNS) disorders, such as the presence of tumours, lesions, gliomas and meningiomas. All the agents are intravascular and extracellular in nature. They are injected intravenously shortly before scanning and distribute within tumours, for example, by passing through a leaky BBB which has been damaged by the particular pathology. An example is shown on the right of Figure 5.47, where the small localized high intensity area on the T_1-weighted image indicates a small tumour in the brain of the patient. The agent remains at an elevated level in the tumour for tens of minutes to a few hours, and then is rapidly cleared through the kidneys since the chelates are highly hydrophilic and do not bind to blood proteins.

Typical patient doses of gadolinium agents are a volume of 10 ml at a concentration of 0.5 M, which results in a concentration in the body of ~0.1 mmol/kg. The greater is the concentration of contrast agent, the shorter the T_1 value. The relationship is given by:

$$\frac{1}{T_1^{CA}} = \frac{1}{T_1} + \alpha_1 C, \tag{5.46}$$

where $T_1{}^{CA}$ is the T_1 of tissue after administration of the contrast agent, T_1 is the pre-adminstration value, and α_1 is the T_1-relaxivity of the contrast agent.

Gd contrast agents are also used in magnetic resonance angiography, covered in Section 5.17. Specifically, a new agent called Gadovist was approved in late 2008. This agent binds strongly but reversibly to human serum albumin in the blood, and so has a much longer half-life in the blood than other Gd-based agents, which are designed to bind weakly: thus Gadovist has primarily a vascular distribution. It is used to study vessel structure in diseases such as peripheral vascular disease, and also to detect arterial stenosis and plaque formation within arteries.

Although Gd-based agents were judged to be completely safe until about 2005, there is increasing evidence that patients with pre-existing kidney disease are a particular concern given the risk of nephrogenic systemic fibrosis (NSF). Only a very small fraction of patients contract this condition, and the mechanism and degree of risk are still currently areas of active research.

5.19.2 Negative contrast agents

The second general class, namely superparamagnetic MRI contrast agents act primarily as negative contrast agents, i.e. they reduce the MR signal in the tissues in which they accumulate. They are used for liver disease, specifically for confirming the presence of liver lesions or focal nodular hyperplasia. These agents consist of small magnetic particles containing iron oxide with a biocompatible coating. Ultra-small superparamagnetic iron oxides (USPIOs) have a core which is less than 30 nm in diameter, whereas superparamagnetic iron oxides (SPIOs) have diameters between 30 and 100 nm. The only agent that is currently approved for worldwide use is Feridex/Endorem with a diameter ~100 nm. A second agent, Resovist is used in the European Union, Australia and Japan, and has a 62 nm diameter core. The recommended intravenous dosage of Feridex is 0.56 milligrams of iron per kg body weight, which is diluted in 100 ml of 5% dextrose solution and given intravenously over 30 minutes. To avoid larger clumps developing, the diluted drug is administered through a 5 micron filter.

Superparamagnetic contrast agents work by causing very strong inhomogeneities in the local magnetic field. Water molecules diffusing through these localized inhomogeneities undergo very fast T_2 and $T_2{}^*$ relaxation, and therefore there is a reduction in signal intensity in the tissues in which the agent accumulates on $T_2{}^*$-weighted gradient-echo or T_2-weighted spin-echo sequences. Small particles are taken up primarily by Kuppfer cells in the liver, but also accumulate in the lymph

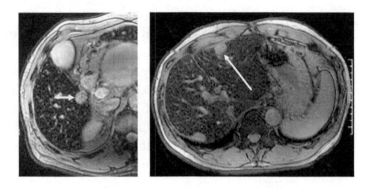

Figure 5.48

Two examples of hepatocellular carcinomas (indicated by the white arrows) imaged after injection of USPIO negative contrast agents. The surrounding liver tissue is dark in the T_2^*-weighted gradient echo imaging sequences, but the carcinomas do not take up the agent and so appear bright relative to the healthy tissue.

nodes, spleen and bone marrow. The particles enter only the healthy Kuppfer cells in the liver and do not accumulate in tumours or other pathological structures. Therefore, these particles reduce the signal intensity from the healthy tissue, with the tumour intensity remaining unaffected as a relatively bright area, as shown in Figure 5.48.

5.20   Image characteristics

As with all imaging modalities, there are trade-offs between image SNR, spatial resolution and CNR. The major factors affecting each of these three parameters are outlined in the following sections.

5.20.1   Signal-to-noise

(i) B_0 field strength. The signal is proportional to the net magnetization, M_0, which is directly proportional to the value of B_0 from Equation (5.10). The signal measured by Faraday induction is directly proportional to the precession frequency from Equation (5.14) and so again proportional to the value of B_0. As seen in Figure 5.28, however, the higher the B_0, the larger the T_1 value and the smaller the image intensity for a given value of TR, Equation (5.34). This latter effect depends, of course, upon the particular tissue and the field strength involved. The value of T_2 is also shorter at higher fields, again with a strong

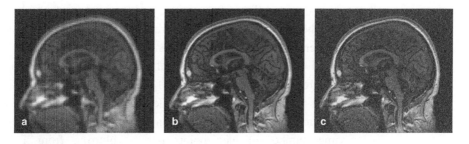

The trade-offs between SNR and spatial resolution. The three images are acquired with identical TR, TE and slice thickness. The image in (a) has a data matrix size of 64×64: the SNR is high, but the image appears 'blocky' with poor spatial resolution. The image in (b) has a matrix size of 128×128: the SNR is still relatively high. In image (c) with a data matrix of 256×256 the image is very 'grainy' due to the poor SNR.

tissue-type dependence: the signal will therefore decrease for a given value of TE. The noise in the image arises primarily from the random voltage induced in the RF coil(s) from the patient, which is proportional to the square-root of the field strength.

(ii) Imaging parameters. Too short a value of TR, too high a value of tip angle, or too long a value of TE reduces the signal intensity from its optimal value. If the image in-plane spatial resolution is doubled from, for example, 1×1 mm to 0.5×0.5 mm, then the SNR per voxel decreases by approximately a factor of 4, assuming all other imaging parameters are kept constant, as shown in Figure 5.49. The total imaging time is also doubled, due to twice the number of phase encoding steps being acquired. The SNR is inversely proportional to the slice thickness, since the number of protons is decreased using a thinner slice. In order to increase the SNR of an image, while maintaining the same spatial resolution, the imaging sequence can be repeated a number of times and the images added together. The MR signal is coherent, but the noise is incoherent, and so the overall SNR increases by the square-root of the number of images: however, the data acquisition time is lengthened by a factor equal to the number of images.

5.20.2 Spatial resolution

The spatial resolution in the three dimensions for most imaging sequences is simply defined by: (i) the slice thickness, (ii) the field-of-view in the phase-encoded dimension divided by the number of phase-encoding steps, and (iii) the field-of-view in the frequency-encoded dimension divided by the number of acquired data points in that dimension. The trade-off between spatial resolution, SNR and total data acquisition time has been outlined in the previous section. It should be noted that, in addition to the three factors outlined previously, single-shot sequences such as EPI can have significantly poorer spatial resolution than multi-shot sequences acquired with the same number of data points due to blurring from T_2^* decay during the sequence.

5.20.3   Contrast-to-noise

Image contrast can be based on differences in proton density, T_1, T_2 or T_2^* relaxation times, or a combination of more than one or all of these parameters. The contrast can be manipulated by appropriate choices of the TR and TE times. Contrast in T_1-weighted sequences decreases with field strength, since the spectral density and therefore T_1 for different tissues approach the same value, as shown in Figure 5.28. For small lesions, the contrast is increased by having high spatial resolution to minimize partial volume effects. However, if the spatial resolution is too high, then the SNR decreases, as shown in Figure 5.50.

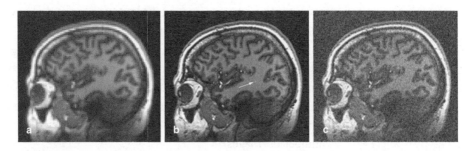

Figure 5.50

The trade-off between CNR, spatial resolution and SNR in MRI. A small hyperintense lesion is visible (white arrow) in image (b) which has a data matrix of 128 × 128. Using a lower data matrix of 64 × 64, image (a) produces a higher SNR, but the spatial resolution is not sufficient to see the lesion. Increasing the spatial resolution by acquiring a 256 × 256 data matrix, image (c), decreases the SNR so that the lesion is again not visible. The optimum spatial resolution for the best CNR in this case is given by image (b).

5.21   Safety considerations – specific absorption rate (SAR)

Associated with any RF magnetic field is a corresponding RF electrical field which produces electric currents in conductive tissues. A key safety consideration in MRI is the power deposition in tissue, quantified via the local and average specific absorption rate (SAR) values, measured in Watts per kilogram. There are strict regulatory guidelines on these values in terms of peak instantaneous and time-averaged values for both local and global regions of interest. The SAR can be calculated from the electric field (E) distributions and is given by:

$$SAR = \frac{\sigma}{2\rho}|E|^2, \qquad (5.47)$$

where ρ is the tissue density and σ the tissue conductivity. The SAR is proportional to the square of the B_1 field multiplied by the time for which the B_1 field is applied, and therefore sequences such as a TSE can result in considerable power deposition within the patient. Every commercial MRI scanner has built-in software and hardware to estimate the SAR for each sequence run, and to adjust the imaging parameters in order to remain within regulatory safety limits.

5.22   Lipid suppression techniques

In only a few clinical applications does the spatial distribution of lipid within a particular organ have important diagnostic information. Otherwise it produces a signal that can mask the pathology which is being detected. Examples include small nodules in the liver and spinal cord, which may be surrounded by a significant signal from lipid. Since lipid has a very short T_1 value and long T_2 value it appears very bright on most images. Fortunately, there are a number of techniques that can be used to minimize the signal from lipid in the image, so-called lipid suppression techniques. Two of these are shown schematically in Figure 5.51. The first is a 'chemical shift selective sequence'. As described in Section 5.6, the protons in lipid resonate at a different frequency from those in water. Therefore, prior to the imaging sequence a 90° frequency-selective RF pulse is applied which tips only the magnetization from the lipid protons into the transverse plane. A gradient is then applied to dephase this magnetization, thus destroying the signal. Now the regular imaging sequence is applied, but since the lipid signal has been completely dephased, it does not produce any signal on the image. The second sequence, shown in Figure 5.51(b), relies on the fact that the T_1 of lipid is much shorter than for most other tissues. A 180° 'inversion pulse' is applied to convert $+M_z$ magnetization into $-M_z$ magnetization for all the protons in the slice. The pulse is turned off and the protons relax back towards equilibrium due to T_1

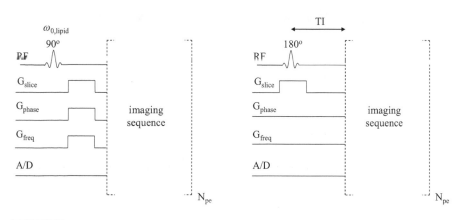

(a) Lipid saturation using frequency-selective excitation. The RF pulse tips only lipid protons into the transverse plane: the magnetization is then rapidly dephased using 'crusher' gradients. The imaging sequence then gives a signal only from the protons in tissue water. (b) An alternative method for lipid suppression. After the 180° pulse, an inversion delay (TI) is used, with the value chosen so that the lipid signal has zero longitudinal magnetization due to T_1 relaxation, at which time the imaging sequence begins.

relaxation. At a specific time, termed the inversion time (TI), after the 180° pulse, the imaging sequence is started. The inversion time is chosen specifically so that the protons in lipid have relaxed back to a value of $M_z = 0$. When the imaging sequence is run, therefore, the slice selective pulse produces no transverse magnetization from the lipid and therefore no signal in the image. These lipid-suppression sequences are called 'inversion recovery' sequences, with the most common clinical acronym being short time inversion recovery (STIR).

5.23 Clinical applications

Almost all parts of the body are imaged in the clinical setting: the brain and spinal cord, the entire musculoskeletal system (shoulder, knee, ankle, and hand), MR mammography, body imaging of the liver, kidneys, urinary tract and prostate, and cardiological applications looking at heart disease. The following applications represent only a small fraction of the total spectrum of clinical protocols.

5.23.1 Neurological applications

MRI can be used to diagnose both acute and chronic neurological diseases, and is the imaging method of choice for intracranial mass lesions such as tumours, with the majority of imaging protocols involving administration of a positive contrast agent.

Many pathological conditions in the brain, such as vasogenic or cytotoxic oedema, result in increased water content, which gives a high signal intensity on T_2-weighted sequences. Oedema is easily seen on T_2-weighted sequences, and has different causes. Interstitial oedema arises from different forms of hydrocephalus, vasogenic oedema arises from breakdown of the BBB in primary and metastatic tumours, and cytotoxic oedema is associated with ischemia.

Tumours located outside the brain (extra-axial tumours), examples of which are meningioma, lymphoma, and schwannoma, are usually benign and after injection of the contrast agent they enhance because of the tumour vascularity. Since they are outside the brain they do not possess a BBB. Intra-axial tumours, such as astrocytoma and glioblastomas, originate within the brain. These also enhance with Gd administration, with high grade tumours generally enhancing more than low grade.

Stroke arises from large vessel occlusion. The cellular sodium/potassium pump fails, leading to cytotoxic oedema. Thrombolytic therapy must be used within the first few hours after stroke and so early detection is key. Early cytotoxic oedema can be detected using diffusion-weighted MRI which is very sensitive to cell swelling. About 20% of strokes come from occlusion of small arteries branching from the major cerebral arteries, and can be visualized as small round lesions in T_2-weighted scans, as well as showing enhancement on contrast agent administration due to disruption of the BBB.

Chronic diseases can either be characterized by specific features such as white matter lesions, in multiple sclerosis for example as shown in Figure 5.52, or more diffuse areas of low intensity which indicate long-term accumulation of iron in areas such as the putamen, a characteristic of Huntington's and Alzheimer's disease. Diagnosis in the latter cases is more difficult than for specific pathologies, since there are a number of other diseases which can lead to similar chronic events, and indeed the normal ageing process results in non-specific white-matter lesions as well as increased iron deposition.

5.23.2 Body applications

Both diffuse and focal liver diseases can be diagnosed using MRI. Scans are normally acquired during a single breath-hold of 10–20 s to avoid image artifacts from respiration. MRI is particularly useful for diagnosing lesions in fatty livers, since these can be obscured in ultrasound and CT. Lesions such as hepatic adenoma enhance strongly after positive contrast administration. Cirrhosis of the liver involves fibrosis which is irreversible, and atrophy in the different lobes is

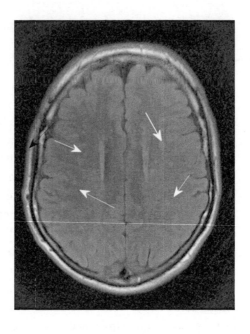

Figure 5.52

Axial image of a subject with white matter lesions (arrows) which can be an early indication of multiple sclerosis.

very common. Cirrhosis also affects blood flow within the liver, and these changes can be seen on TOF angiograms with or without contrast agent administration. Diseases such as haemochromatosis and haemolytic anaemia can be associated with cirrhosis. Iron overload is seen as a very low signal on T_2-weighted sequences, with lipid and muscle effectively acting as internal references in terms of signal intensity.

Metastases are the most common form of liver tumours, and can be diagnosed using contrast agent injection. Images must be acquired very rapidly after injection of the agent. Liver cysts can be differentiated from tumours by the fact that they do not enhance. Hemangiomas are benign focal liver lesions and, being filled with water, give low signal intensity on T_1-weighted sequences and high signal intensity on T_2-weighted sequences. Larger hemangiomas typically enhance first on the periphery of the structure, and then slowly the enhancement 'fills in' the entire structure, as shown in Figure 5.53(b).

5.23.3 Musculoskeletal applications

MRI can produce high quality images of the entire musculoskeletal (MSK) system. One application is in the evaluation of cartilage integrity in the knee, with

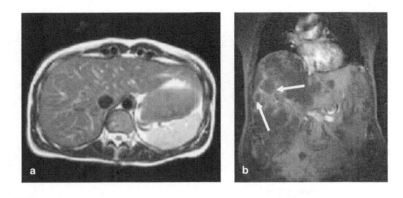

(a) Axial slice showing the liver filling essentially the entire field-of-view of the image. (b) Coronal image acquired after administration of a positive contrast agent, showing inhomogeneous enhancement of a hemangioma.

degradation being associated with diseases such as rheumatoid- and osteo-arthritis. The cartilage shows up as a well-defined area of high signal intensity just below the knee cap, as shown in Figure 5.54 (a). Other areas of MSK imaging include the hand/wrist, shown in Figure 5.54(b), which can also be affected by different forms of arthritis, and the ankle. Assessment of diseases of the spinal cord, Figure 5.54(c), can be classified into neurological, oncological or MSK. Degenerative diseases of the spinal cord are very commonly diagnosed using MRI. On T_2-weighted images, normal intervertebral discs are bright: degnerative disc disease reduces the water content of the discs which therefore become darker. Tumours in the spinal cord itself can be detected via enhancement after administration of positive contrast agent.

5.23.4 Cardiology applications

In all cardiac scans gating of data acquisition to the cardiac cycle (using electro-cardiogram measurements with MRI-compatible equipment) is necessary to reduce the artifacts associated with heart motion. In studies of ischemic heart disease, MRI is used to visualize myocardial infarcts which have a high intensity on T_2-weighted sequences due to myocardial oedema. Positive contrast enhancement is also indicative of a recent infarct. Indirect measurements of cardiac wall thinning also provide evidence of a local infarct. There is normally excellent contrast between blood in the myocardium (which is bright) and the myocardial wall itself, as shown in Figure 5.55(a). The left ventricular volume and ejection fraction are very important measures of heart function, and both can be measured using MRI. In addition, using spin-tagging techniques, the complex motion of the

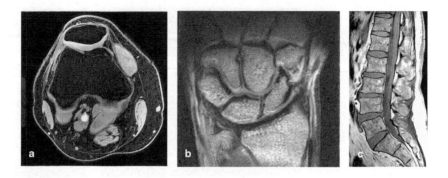

Figure 5.54

(a) Axial image of the knee, showing a bright area of patellar cartilage and below it the 'mottled' pattern corresponding to trabecular bone structure. (b) Sagittal view of the hand, again showing cartilage and trabecular bone structures. (c) Sagittal image of the spinal cord and vertebral column.

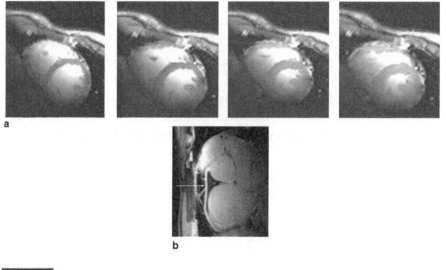

Figure 5.55

(a) A slice through the heart at four stages of the cardiac cycle, showing the expansion and contraction of the myocardium (low gray signal), with blood showing as a bright signal. (b) Image of the left coronary artery in a subject, shown by the arrow.

heart wall during systole and diastole can be investigated for abnormalities. Morphological changes associated with different types of cardiomyopathy can also be seen using MRI.

Left anterior descending coronary artery disease is one of the most common causes of heart attacks, and stenoses of the coronary arteries can be assessed using angiographic techniques: an example is shown in Figure 5.55(b).

Exercises

Basics (Sections 5.2–5.4)

5.1 Assuming that there are 6.7×10^{22} protons in a cubic centimeter of water, what is the magnetization contained within this volume at a magnetic field strength of 3 Tesla?

5.2 Using classical mechanics, show that the effect of an RF pulse applied around the x-axis is to rotate z-magnetization towards the y-axis.

5.3 Show schematically the separate effects of: (i) a 90_x°, (ii) a 180_x°, (iii) a 270_x°, and (iv) a 360_x° pulse on thermal equilibrium magnetization using the vector model.

5.4 What is the effect of changing the orientation of the RF coil so that it produces a pulse about the z-axis?

5.5 Calculate the effects of the following pulse sequences on thermal equilibrium magnetization. The final answer should include x-, y-, and z-components of magnetization.

a) 90°_x (a pulse with tip angle 90°, applied about the x-axis).

b) 80°_x.

c) $90^\circ_x \, 90^\circ_y$ (the second 90° pulse is applied immediately after the first).

T_1 and T_2 relaxation times

5.6 Answer true or false with one or two sentences of explanation:

a) recovery of magnetization along the z-axis after a 90° pulse does not necessarily result in loss of magnetization from the xy-plane;

b) a static magnetic field B_0 that is homogeneous results in a free induction decay which persists for a long time;

c) a short tissue T_1 indicates a slow spin-lattice relaxation process.

5.7 Write an expression for the M_z magnetization as a function of time after a 180° pulse. After what time is the M_z component zero? Plot the magnetization after instead applying a 135° pulse.

5.8 The hydrogen nuclei in the body are found mainly in lipid and water. The T_2 value of lipid was measured to be 100 ms, and that of water to be 500 ms. In a spin-echo experiment, calculate the delay between the 90° pulse and the 180° pulse which maximizes the difference in signal intensities between the lipid and water. Assume that the total number of lipid protons is the same as the total number of water protons.

MRI and basic imaging sequences

5.9 The operator wishes to acquire an oblique slice shown by the orientation of the white bar in Figure 5.56 (a). Draw the gradient echo imaging sequence that would be run to acquire such an image.

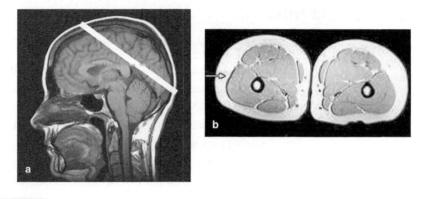

(a) See Exercise 5.9, (b) See Exercise 5.14.

5.10 A multi-slice spin-echo imaging sequence is run with the following parameters: a 256×256 data matrix, TR is 2 seconds, TE is 20 ms, and ten slices are acquired. How long does the MRI scan take to complete?

5.11 Derive the value of the Ernst angle given in Equation (5.35).

5.12 Given a maximum magnetic field gradient of 40 mT/m, how homogeneous must the static magnetic field be (in parts per million) to enable a spatial resolution of 1 mm to be acquired?

5.13 Assume that in a Fourier imaging experiment, the desired phase-encoding gradients are $G_n = n\Delta G_0$. What will happen to the reconstructed image if the gradient system malfunctions such that the effective gradients applied are: $G_n = n(\Delta G_0/2)$?

5.14 In the image shown in Figure 5.56 (b), acquired using a standard spin-echo sequence, the bright signal corresponds to lipid and the lower intensity signal to water. The lipid and water signals appear spatially shifted with respect to one another.

   (i) Given the facts above, which of the left/right or up/down dimensions corresponds to the frequency encoding direction, and which to the phase encoding direction? Explain your answer fully.

  (ii) The image is acquired at a field strength of 3 Tesla, and the black band in the image is 3 pixels wide. If the total image data size is 256×256, what is the overall data acquisition bandwidth? The image field-of-view is 5×5 cm: what is the strength of the frequency encoding gradient?

 (iii) If the frequency encoding gradient were increased by a factor of 3, what effect would this have on the imaging artifact?

5.15 Use the concept of avoiding signal aliasing to derive the image field-of-view in the phase encoding dimension. The answer should include the value of the

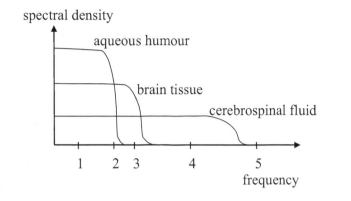

spectral density

aqueous humour

brain tissue

cerebrospinal fluid

1 2 3 4 5

frequency

Figure 5.57

See Exercise 5.17.

incremental phase encoding gradient step, the length of time that the gradient is applied for, and any relevant physical constants.

Tissue relaxation times

5.16 (a) Plot qualitatively the dependence of T_1 on the strength of the applied magnetic field for a mobile, an intermediate and a viscous liquid.

(b) Plot qualitatively the variation in T_1 as a function of the mobility of a liquid.

5.17 For the five frequencies (1–5) shown in Figure 5.57, state the order of the T_1 values, e.g. T_1(brain) $> T_1$ (CSF) $> T_1$ (aqueous humour). Where possible, do the same for the T_2 values.

Relaxation weighted imaging sequences

5.18 Choose the correct option from (a)-(e) and explain why this is your choice. The maximum MR signal is obtained by using:

(a) 90° RF pulse, short TE, and short TR;

(b) 45° RF pulse, short TE, and short TR;

(c) 90° RF pulse, short TE, and long TR;

(d) 90° RF pulse, long TE, and short TR;

(e) 45° RF pulse, long TE, and short TR.

5.19 Choose the correct option from (a)-(e) and explain why this is your choice. Water in tendons is bound very strongly and cannot diffuse freely. It produces very low MR signal intensity because:

(a) T_1 is too short;

(b) T_2 is too short;

(c) T_2^* is very long;

(d) T_2 is longer than T_1;

(e) T_2^* is longer than T_2.

5.20 A brain tumour has a lower concentration of water than surrounding healthy tissue. The T_1 value of the protons in the tumour is shorter than that of the protons in healthy tissue, but the T_2 value of the tumour protons is longer. Which kind of weighting should be introduced into the imaging sequence in order to ensure that there is contrast between the tumour and healthy tissue? If a large concentration of superparamagnetic contrast agent is injected and accumulates in the tumour only, which kind of weighting would now be optimal?

5.21 A region of the brain to be imaged contains areas corresponding to tumour, normal brain and lipid. The relevant MRI parameters are:

$$\rho(\text{tumour}) = \rho(\text{lipid}) > \rho(\text{brain})$$
$$T_1(\text{lipid}) > T_1(\text{tumour}) > T_1(\text{brain})$$
$$T_2(\text{lipid}) > T_2(\text{tumour}) > T_2(\text{brain}).$$

Which type of weighted spin-echo sequence should be run in order to get contrast between the three different tissues. Explain your reasoning, including why the other two types of weighting would not work.

5.22 Three MRIs of the brain are acquired using identical parameters except for the TR and TE times. Three tumours (upper, middle and lower) are seen in one of the images but not in the other two, as shown in Figure 5.58. If the T_1 values for all the tissues (tumours and brain) are less than 2 s, and the T_2 values are all greater than 80 ms, describe the *relative* values of proton density, T_1 and T_2 of brain tissue and the three tumours.

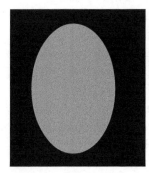 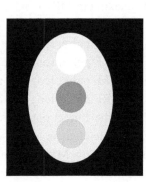 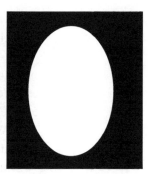

TR=0.5 s, TE=80 ms   TR=0.5 s, TE=1 ms   TR=10 s, TE=1 ms

See Exercise 5.22.

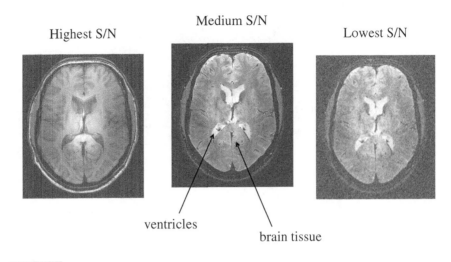

Highest S/N   Medium S/N   Lowest S/N

ventricles   brain tissue

Figure 5.59

See Exercise 5.23.

5.23 Three images are shown in Figure 5.59: the scaling in each image is different and is normalized to the same maximum value. The imaging parameters are TR = 2000 ms, TE = 20 ms for one image, TR = 750 ms, TE = 80 ms for another, and TR = 2000 ms, TE = 80 ms for the final one.

(i) Assign each image to the appropriate TR and TE values.

(ii) Based on your answer, do the ventricles have a higher or lower T_1 value than brain tissue? What is the corresponding answer for T_2?

5.24 The T_1-weighted image in Figure 5.60 represents a slice through the abdomen, with signals coming from liver, kidney, tumour and lipid. Given the following information:

$$\rho(\text{liver}) = \rho(\text{kidney}) < \rho(\text{lipid}) < \rho(\text{tumour})$$

and the spectral density plot shown below:

(a) Determine at which frequency (ω_1, ω_2, ω_3 or ω_4) the image was acquired, and give your reasons.

(b) At which of these frequencies (ω_1, ω_2, ω_3 or ω_4) would the relative signal intensities of the four tissues be reversed, i.e. the highest becomes lowest and vice-versa?

k-space

5.25 For a spiral k-space trajectory shown in Figure 5.61 (a), draw the gradient waveforms for the x- and y-gradients.

5.26 Design an EPI pulse sequence that gives the square spiral k-space trajectory shown in Figure 5.61 (b).

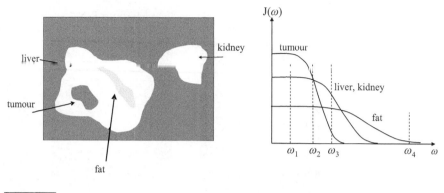

Figure 5.60

See Exercise 5.24.

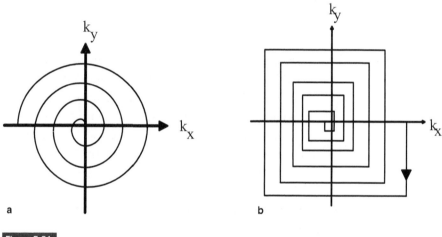

a   b

Figure 5.61.

See Exercises 5.25 and 5.26.

MR contrast agents

5.27 For Gd-DTPA the value of α_1 is approximately 5 mM^{-1} s^{-1}. Assuming that a small white matter lesion has a T_1 of 1.2 s at 3 Tesla, and that the concentration of Gd-chelate inside the lesion is 2 mM, what is the T_1 of the lesion post-administration of the contrast agent. If a T_1-weighted gradient echo sequence is run with a TR of 100 ms and a tip angle of 10°, how much is the signal increased post-administration?

5.28 Assuming a T_1 value of tissue and blood of 1 s, calculate the $T_{1(eff)}$ as a function of blood velocity of 5 cm/s for a slice thickness of 5 mm. Using a TR of 50 ms and a tip angle of 60°, what are the relative signal

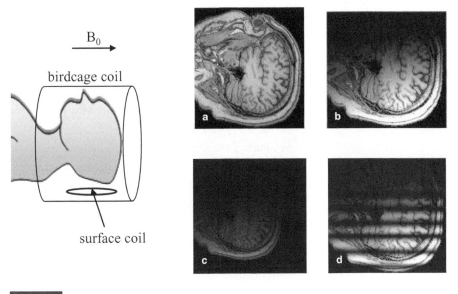

B_0

birdcage coil

surface coil

Figure 5.62

See Exercise 5.29.

intensities from blood and stationary tissue? If a contrast agent is added to the blood so that the T_1 of blood is reduced to 200 ms, what are the relative values?

MRI instrumentation

5.29 A brain MRI is being performed on a patient. Two RF coils are available to obtain the images, a birdcage coil and a surface coil as shown in Figure 5.62. Each can be used to transmit the RF pulses, receive the signal, or both transmit and receive. Images A to D correspond to different combinations of the two coils used in transmit, receive or both transmit and receive mode. State, with reasons, which combination of transmit and receive (i.e. Image A, surface coil transmit, birdcage coil receive) on which coils are used for the four images A-D.

5.30 Draw two electrical circuits which could be used as analogues to Figure 5.37 for the transmit RF coil.

Lipid suppression

5.31 If the lipid T_1 value is 360 ms and the value for muscle is 1420 ms, calculate the inversion time necessary to null the signal from lipid. What percentage of the signal from tissue is observed using this inversion time?

5.32 Explain why inversion recovery sequences for lipid suppression are not a good choice after positive contrast agent administration.

Review

5.33 Explain whether each of the following statements is true or false, with one or two sentences of explanation.

(a) Protons precessing at a higher frequency relax back to equilibrium faster and so have a shorter T_1 relaxation time.

(b) A higher strength of the RF field from the RF coil means that the duration of the 90° pulse decreases.

(c) A longer T_1 relaxation time means that the voltage induced in the RF coil lasts longer and so a larger MRI signal is achieved.

(d) One line of k-space data acquired for each value of the phase encoding gradient corresponds to one line of the image.

(e) All other parameters being equal, a longer RF pulse in a spin-echo imaging sequence results in a lower signal-to-noise.

(f) At very high magnetic fields the T_1 values of all tissues approach the same value.

References

[1] Bloch F. Nuclear induction. *Physical Review* 1946;**70**(7–8), 460–74.

[2] Lauterbur PC. Image formation by induced local interactions – examples employing nuclear magnetic-resonance. *Nature* 1973;**242**(5394), 190–1.

[3] Kumar A, Welti D and Ernst RR. Nmr Fourier Zeugmatography. *J Magn Reson* 1975;**18**(1), 69–83.

[4] Edelstein WA, Hutchison JMS, Johnson G and Redpath T. Spin warp Nmr imaging and applications to human whole-body imaging. *Physics in Medicine and Biology* 1980;**25**(4), 751–6.

[5] Ljunggren S. A simple graphical representation of Fourier-based imaging methods. *J Magn Reson* 1983;**54**(2), 338–43.

[6] Hahn EL. Spin echoes. *Physical Review* 1950;**80**(4), 580–94.

[7] Hedeen RA and Edelstein WA. Characterization and prediction of gradient acoustic noise in MR imagers. *Magn Reson Med* 1997;**37**(1), 7–10.

[8] Turner R. Gradient coil design – A review of methods. *Magnetic Resonance Imaging* 1993;**11**(7), 903–20.

[9] Chapman BLW and Mansfield P. Quiet gradient coils – active acoustically and magnetically screened distributed transverse gradient designs. *Measurement Science & Technology* 1995;**6**(4), 349–54.

[10] Mansfield P and Chapman B. Active magnetic screening of gradient coils in Nmr imaging. *J Magn Reson* 1986 Feb 15;**66**(3), 573–6.

[11] Hayes CE, Edelstein WA, Schenck JF, Mueller OM and Eash M. An efficient, highly homogeneous radiofrequency coil for whole-body Nmr imaging at 1.5-T. *J Magn Reson* 1985;**63**(3), 622–8.

[12] Roemer PB, Edelstein WA, Hayes CE, Souza SP and Mueller OM. The NMR phased array. *Magn Reson Med* 1990 Nov;**16**(2), 192–225.

[13] Edelstein WA, Hardy CJ and Mueller OM. Electronic decoupling of surface-coil receivers for Nmr imaging and spectroscopy. *J Magn Reson* 1986 Mar;**67**(1), 156–61.

[14] Carlson JW and Minemura T. Imaging time reduction through multiple receiver coil data acquisition and image reconstruction. *Magn Reson Med* 1993;**29**(5), 681–7.

[15] Sodickson DK and Manning WJ. Simultaneous acquisition of spatial harmonics (SMASH): fast imaging with radiofrequency coil arrays. *Magn Reson Med* 1997 Oct;**38**(4), 591–603.

[16] Pruessmann KP, Weiger M, Scheidegger MB and Boesiger P. SENSE: sensitivity encoding for fast MRI. *Magn Reson Med* 1999 Nov;**42**(5), 952–62.

[17] Griswold MA, Jakob PM, Heidemann RM *et al*. Generalized autocalibrating partially parallel acquisitions (GRAPPA). *Magn Reson Med* 2002;**47**(6), 1202–10.

[18] Mansfield P. Multi-planar image-formation using Nmr spin echoes. *Journal of Physics C-Solid State Physics* 1977;**10**(3), L55–L58.

[19] Hennig J, Nauerth A and Friedburg H. RARE imaging: a fast imaging method for clinical MR. *Magn Reson Med* 1986 Dec;**3**(6), 823–33.

[20] Crooks LE, Mills CM, Davis PL, *et al*. Visualization of cerebral and vascular abnormalities by NMR imaging. The effects of imaging parameters on contrast. *Radiology* 1982 Sep;**144**(4), 843–52.

[21] Ogawa S, Lee TM, Kay AR and Tank DW. Brain magnetic resonance imaging with contrast dependent on blood oxygenation. *Proc Natl Acad Sci U S A* 1990 Dec;**87**(24), 9868–72.

Index